Caffeine for the Sustainment of Mental Task Performance

Formulations for Military Operations

Committee on Military Nutrition Research

Food and Nutrition Board

INSTITUTE OF MEDICINE

NATIONAL ACADEMY PRESS
Washington, D.C.

NATIONAL ACADEMY PRESS • 2101 Constitution Avenue, NW • Washington, DC 20418

NOTICE: The project that is the subject of this report was approved by the Governing Board of the National Research Council, whose members are drawn from the councils of the National Academy of Sciences, the National Academy of Engineering, and the Institute of Medicine. The members of the committee responsible for the report were chosen for their special competences and with regard for appropriate balance.

Support for this project was provided by the U.S. Department of the Army, Army Medical Research and Materiel Command through grant No. DAMD17-94-J-4046 and grant No. DAMD17-99-1-9478. The U.S. Army Medical Research Acquisition Activity, 820 Chandler Street, Fort Detrick, MD 21702-5014, is the awarding and administering acquisition office. The views presented in this publication are those of the Committee on Military Nutrition Research and do not necessarily reflect the position or policy of the government, and no official endorsement should be inferred.

International Standard Book Number 0-309-08258-7
Library of Congress Control Number 2001097708

This report is available for sale from the National Academy Press, 2101 Constitution Avenue, N.W., Box 285, Washington, DC 20055; call (800) 624-6242 or (202) 334-3313 (in the Washington metropolitan area), or visit the NAP's on-line bookstore at **http://www.nap.edu**.

For more information about the Institute of Medicine and the Food and Nutrition Board, visit the IOM and FNB home pages at **http://www.iom/** and **http://www.iom/fnb/**.

Copyright 2001 by the National Academy of Sciences. All rights reserved.

Printed in the United States of America.

Knowing is not enough; we must apply.
Willing is not enough; we must do.
—Goethe

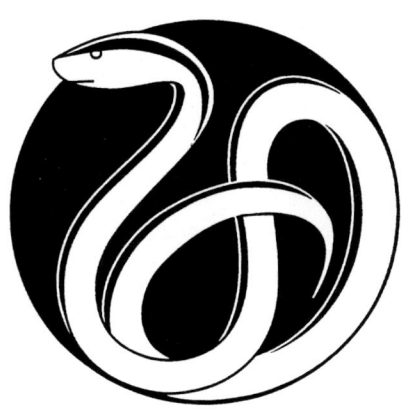

INSTITUTE OF MEDICINE

Shaping the Future for Health

THE NATIONAL ACADEMIES

National Academy of Sciences
National Academy of Engineering
Institute of Medicine
National Research Council

The **National Academy of Sciences** is a private, nonprofit, self-perpetuating society of distinguished scholars engaged in scientific and engineering research, dedicated to the furtherance of science and technology and to their use for the general welfare. Upon the authority of the charter granted to it by the Congress in 1863, the Academy has a mandate that requires it to advise the federal government on scientific and technical matters. Dr. Bruce M. Alberts is president of the National Academy of Sciences.

The **National Academy of Engineering** was established in 1964, under the charter of the National Academy of Sciences, as a parallel organization of outstanding engineers. It is autonomous in its administration and in the selection of its members, sharing with the National Academy of Sciences the responsibility for advising the federal government. The National Academy of Engineering also sponsors engineering programs aimed at meeting national needs, encourages education and research, and recognizes the superior achievements of engineers. Dr. Wm. A. Wulf is president of the National Academy of Engineering.

The **Institute of Medicine** was established in 1970 by the National Academy of Sciences to secure the services of eminent members of appropriate professions in the examination of policy matters pertaining to the health of the public. The Institute acts under the responsibility given to the National Academy of Sciences by its congressional charter to be an adviser to the federal government and, upon its own initiative, to identify issues of medical care, research, and education. Dr. Kenneth I. Shine is president of the Institute of Medicine.

The **National Research Council** was organized by the National Academy of Sciences in 1916 to associate the broad community of science and technology with the Academy's purposes of furthering knowledge and advising the federal government. Functioning in accordance with general policies determined by the Academy, the Council has become the principal operating agency of both the National Academy of Sciences and the National Academy of Engineering in providing services to the government, the public, and the scientific and engineering communities. The Council is administered jointly by both Academies and the Institute of Medicine. Dr. Bruce M. Alberts and Dr. Wm. A. Wulf are chairman and vice chairman, respectively, of the National Research Council.

COMMITTEE ON MILITARY NUTRITION RESEARCH

JOHN E. VANDERVEEN *(Chair)*, San Antonio, Texas
LAWRENCE E. ARMSTRONG, Departments of Physiology and Neurobiology, and Exercise Science, University of Connecticut, Storrs
GAIL E. BUTTERFIELD *(deceased)*, Nutrition Studies, Palo Alto Veterans Affairs Health Care System and Program in Human Biology, Stanford University, Palo Alto, California
WANDA L. CHENOWETH, Department of Food Science and Human Nutrition, Michigan State University, East Lansing
JOHANNA T. DWYER, Frances Stern Nutrition Center, New England Medical Center Hospital and Departments of Medicine and Community Health, Tufts Medical School and School of Nutrition Science and Policy, Boston, Massachusetts
JOHN D. FERNSTROM, Department of Psychiatry, Pharmacology, and Neuroscience, University of Pittsburgh School of Medicine, Pennsylvania
ROBIN B. KANAREK, Department of Psychology, Tufts University, Boston, Massachusetts
ORVILLE A. LEVANDER, Nutrient Requirements and Functions Laboratory, U.S. Department of Agriculture Beltsville Human Nutrition Research Center, Beltsville, Maryland
ESTHER M. STERNBERG, Neuroendocrine Immunology and Behavior Section, National Institute of Mental Health, Bethesda, Maryland

U.S. Army Grant Representative
LTC KARL E. FRIEDL, U.S. Army, Military Operational Medicine Research Program, U.S. Army Medical Research and Materiel Command, Fort Detrick, Frederick, Maryland

Staff
MARY I. POOS, Study Director
TAZIMA A. DAVIS, Senior Project Assistant (from September 18, 2000)
KARAH NAZOR, Project Assistant (through July 28, 2000)

FOOD AND NUTRITION BOARD

CUTBERTO GARZA (*Chair*), Division of Nutrition, Cornell University, Ithaca, New York
LARRY R. BEUCHAT, Center for Food Safety and Quality Enhancement, University of Georgia, Griffin
BENJAMIN CABALLERO, Center for Human Nutrition, The Johns Hopkins School of Hygiene and Public Health, Baltimore, Maryland
ROBERT J. COUSINS, Center for Nutritional Sciences, University of Florida, Gainesville
SHIRIKI KUMANYIKA, Center for Clinical Epidemiology and Biostatistics, University of Pennsylvania School of Medicine, Philadelphia
ALFRED H. MERRILL, JR., Department of Biochemistry, Emory Center for Nutrition and Health Sciences, Emory University, Atlanta, Georgia
LYNN PARKER, Child Nutrition Programs and Nutrition Policy, Food Research and Action Center, Washington, D.C.
ROSS L. PRENTICE, Division of Public Health Sciences, Fred Hutchinson Cancer Research Center, Seattle, Washington
A. CATHERINE ROSS, Nutrition Department, The Pennsylvania State University, University Park
ROBERT M. RUSSELL, Jean Mayer U.S. Department of Agriculture Human Nutrition Research Center on Aging, Tufts University, Boston, Massachusetts
BARBARA O. SCHNEEMAN, Department of Nutrition, University of California at Davis
ROBERT E. SMITH, R.E. Smith Consulting, Inc., Newport, Vermont
VIRGINIA A. STALLINGS, Division of Gastroenterology and Nutrition, The Children's Hospital of Philadelphia, Pennsylvania
STEVE L. TAYLOR, Department of Food Science and Technology and Food Processing Center, University of Nebraska, Lincoln
BARRY L. ZOUMAS, Department of Agricultural Economics and Rural Sociology, The Pennsylvania State University, University Park

Staff
ALLISON A. YATES, Director
LINDA MEYERS, Deputy Director
GAIL SPEARS, Staff Editor
GEORGE YORK, Administrative Assistant
GARY WALKER, Financial Associate

Dedication

The Committee on Military Nutrition Research dedicates this report to the late Gail Butterfield, a diligent and enthusiastic member of the committee who made invaluable contributions to this study and numerous other studies during her six years of service. Her unique background in nutrition and physiology was a special asset to the committee's work. She was dedicated to contributing to the health and nutritional well-being of America's military personnel, both active-duty members and veterans.

Reviewers

This report has been reviewed in draft form by individuals chosen for their diverse perspectives and technical expertise, in accordance with procedures approved by the National Research Council's Report Review Committee. The purpose of this independent review is to provide candid and critical comments that will assist the institution in making its published report as sound as possible and to ensure that the report meets institutional standards for objectivity, evidence, and responsiveness to the study charge. The review comments and draft manuscript remain confidential to protect the integrity of the deliberative process. We wish to thank the following individuals for their review of this report:

E. Wayne Askew, University of Utah
Fergus M. Clydesdale, University of Massachusetts
Joseph T. Coyle, Harvard Medical School
David Dinges, University of Pennsylvania School of Medicine
Harold Goforth, Point Loma College
Steven R. Hursh, Science Applications International Corporation

Although the reviewers listed above have provided many constructive comments and suggestions, they were not asked to endorse the conclusions or recommendations nor did they see the final draft of the report before its release. The review of this report was overseen by Catherine E. Woteki, University of Maryland at College Park, appointed by the Institute of Medicine, who was responsible for making certain that an independent examination of this report was carried out in accordance with institutional procedures and that all review comments were carefully considered. Responsibility for the final content of this report rests entirely with the authoring committee and the institution.

Preface

This publication is the latest in a series of reports prepared by the Committee on Military Nutrition Research (CMNR) of the Food and Nutrition Board (FNB), Institute of Medicine, National Academies. Other reports in the series have included such issues as food components to enhance performance; nutritional needs in hot, cold, and high-altitude environments; body composition and physical performance; nutrition and physical performance; cognitive testing methodology; fluid replacement and heat stress; and antioxidants and oxidative stress. These reports are part of the response that the CMNR provides to the commander of the U.S. Army Medical Research and Materiel Command (USAMRMC) regarding issues brought to the committee by the Military Operational Medicine Research Program at Fort Detrick, Maryland, and the Military Nutrition Division of the U.S. Army Research Institute of Environmental Medicine at Natick, Massachusetts. Typically, reports in this series review the scientific background of an issue, and provide direct responses to questions posed by USAMRMC and specific recommendations from CMNR.

HISTORY OF THE COMMITTEE

The CMNR was established in October 1982, following a request by the assistant surgeon general of the Army that the Board on Military Supplies of the National Academy of Sciences set up a special committee. The purpose of this committee was to advise the U.S. Department of Defense on the need for and conduct of nutrition research and related issues. The CMNR was transferred to the FNB in 1983. The CMNR's current tasks are as follows:

- to identify nutritional factors that may critically influence the physical and mental performance of military personnel under all environmental extremes;
- to identify deficiencies in the existing database;

- to recommend research to remedy these deficiencies as well as approaches for studying the relationship of diet to physical and mental performance; and
- to review and advise on standards for military feeding systems.

Within this context, the CMNR was asked to focus on nutrient requirements for performance during operational missions rather than requirements for military personnel in garrison (the latter were judged to be not significantly different from those of the civilian population).

Although the membership of the committee has changed periodically, the disciplines represented consistently have included human nutrition, nutritional biochemistry, performance physiology, food science, and psychology. For issues that require broader expertise than exists within the committee, the CMNR has convened workshops or utilized consultants. The workshops provide additional state-of-the-art scientific information and informed opinion for the consideration of the committee.

ORGANIZATION OF THIS REPORT

Chapter 1 of this report provides background information on the military interest in caffeine and the history of its use, and Chapter 2 briefly reviews caffeine metabolism and pharmacology. Chapters 3 through 6 review the recent scientific literature organized around the Army's task questions of efficacy, safety, formulations, dosage, ethical considerations, and alternatives. The CMNR's summary responses to questions, conclusions, and recommendations are presented in Chapter 7. The workshop agenda and abstracts are presented in Appendix A. Appendix B contains CMNR recommendations concerning caffeine from the report, *Food Components to Enhance Performance* (IOM, 1994). Biographical sketches of CMNR members and the workshop speakers are given in Appendix C. Speakers invited to the workshop were also requested to submit a brief list of selected background papers. Their recommended readings, relevant citations collected by CMNR staff prior to the workshop, and citations from each chapter are included in the references.

ACKNOWLEDGMENTS

It is my pleasure as chairman of the CMNR to acknowledge the contributions of the FNB staff. Their dedication in the planning and organization of the workshop and in editing this report made it possible for the committee to provide an in-depth response to the Army's request. In particular, I wish to acknowledge the superior efforts of Mary I. Poos, the staff officer for the CMNR. She worked diligently with committee members in securing the expert panel of speakers and organizing the program for the workshop into coherent sessions.

She also conducted extensive reviews and summaries of the scientific literature and performed major edits of the report to ensure clarity and accuracy.

I also wish to commend the workshop speakers for their excellent contributions in preparing abstracts and participating through their presentations and discussions at the workshop. Their willingness to take time from very busy schedules to prepare and deliver outstanding presentations made it possible for the committee to conduct the review and prepare this report. Their thoughtful responses to CMNR members' and workshop participants' questions also contributed immeasurably to the quality of the review. It would be neglectful not to mention the many experts who attended this open meeting at their own initiative and expense. Their questions and comments contributed in no small measure to broadening the exchange of scientific information.

I express my deepest appreciation to the members of the CMNR who participated extensively during the workshop and in discussions and preparation of the summary and recommendations in this report. I continue to be stimulated by the committee's dedication and willing contribution of time and expertise to the activities of the CMNR. I thank all of you for your continuing contributions to this program.

JOHN E. VANDERVEEN, *Chair*
Committee on Military Nutrition Research

Contents

EXECUTIVE SUMMARY 1
    Background, 2
    The Committee's Task, 2
    Methods, 3
    Caffeine Use, 4
    Caffeine Metabolism, 4
    Response to Military Questions, 6

1   BASIC CONCEPTS 17
    Military Interest in Caffeine, 17
    History of Caffeine Use, 19
    The Committee's Task, 20

2   PHARMACOLOGY OF CAFFEINE 25
    Absorption, Distribution, and Metabolism, 26
    Factors Affecting Caffeine Metabolism, 28
    Physiological Effects, 29
    Summary, 31

3   EFFICACY OF CAFFEINE 33
    Physical Performance, 33
    Cognitive Function and Alertness, 37
    Compensation of Sleep Deprivation Impairments, 40
    Summary, 44

4   SAFETY OF CAFFEINE USAGE 47
    Caffeine and Cardiovascular Disease Risk, 49
    Caffeine Effects on Reproduction, 52
    Caffeine Effects on Bone Mineral Density, 54
    Caffeine Effects on Fluid Homeostasis, 55

Detrimental Effects of High Doses of Caffeine, 56
Summary, 59

5 DOSES AND DELIVERY MECHANISMS 61
   Optimum Caffeine Dosage, 61
   Caffeine Delivery Mechanisms, 63
   Summary, 65

6 SPECIAL CONSIDERATIONS 67
   Education and Training Issues, 68
   Labeling, 68
   Ethical Considerations, 69
   Alternatives to Caffeine for Maintenance of Cognitive
      Performance, 69
   Summary, 77

7 RESPONSE TO MILITARY QUESTIONS, CONCLUSIONS,
   AND RECOMMENDATIONS 79
   Additional Research Recommendations, 96

REFERENCES 97

APPENDIXES

   A Workshop Agenda and Abstracts, 115
   B Previous Recommendations on Caffeine from the Committee on
      Military Nutrition Research, 143
   C Biographical Sketches, 147

Executive Summary

The goal of any employer, regardless of the field of endeavor, is optimal job performance without compromising the health and well-being of the worker. Intermittent or prolonged physiological and psychological stressors that employees bring to the workplace have an impact not only on their own performance but also on those with whom they work and interact. These stressors are compounded by the physical and mental stressors of the job itself. Military personnel in combat settings endure highly unpredictable timing and types of stressors, both personal and job-related, as well as situations that require continuing vigilance for extended periods of time.

Changes in military operations over the last 50 years have required continued assessment and adoption of technologies that will sustain or enhance physical and cognitive performance of the individual service member. This urgency in maintaining and enhancing performance is fostered by increased reliance on the individual's cognitive skills in the operation and maintenance of complex military equipment in an increasing variety of environmental conditions. Today's military relies heavily on the use of computer-controlled systems that require highly trained and alert individuals. There is also greater reliance on rapid mobility to enable deployment at any time to achieve the nation's military objectives. The urgency to maintain and enhance performance is driven by personnel reductions and shortfalls in recruitment goals—resulting in the need to have the individual perform for longer periods of time with less sleep, shorter transition times, less recovery time between missions, and less reliance on traditional logistical support.

These scenarios can have severe impacts on the individual's level of fatigue, alertness, response time, mood, judgment, reliability in decision making, and other cognitive skills. Increased likelihood of decrements in cognitive function coincides with greater dependence on the individual's performance, and both have a profound impact on the success or failure of a mission.

BACKGROUND

At the request of the U.S. Army Medical Research and Materiel Command (USAMRMC) in 1992, the Committee on Military Nutrition Research (CMNR) of the Institute of Medicine's Food and Nutrition Board reviewed the scientific literature, held a workshop, and produced a report on *Food Components to Enhance Performance* (IOM, 1994). In that report the CMNR recommended that the military pursue additional research on the mechanisms of effects of caffeine on cognitive performance, mood, and alertness, focusing on maximizing positive effects when performance is already degraded.

Specifically, the committee recommended:

> Caffeine definitely should be considered in developing performance-enhancing rations or ration components. Caffeine is safe as a component of food at doses required to overcome sleep deprivation and has been included in diets in coffee and many soft drinks. Since many soldiers may not normally drink coffee, a mechanism for including caffeine in another ration component—that can be selectively used when the situation requires—should be evaluated. It appears that doses of 300–600 mg/70 kg person will achieve the desired stimulus in those not habituated to caffeine; additional research needs to be conducted to determine the effects of this level of caffeine in those with higher habitual intakes. (IOM, 1994, p. 50)

THE COMMITTEE'S TASK

Recent surveys indicate that more than 90 percent of the military population consumes caffeine at some level on a daily basis. Typically, older personnel consume more caffeine than younger ones, and males consume slightly more than females. The majority of caffeine (approximately 70 percent) is consumed as coffee, 23 percent as soda, 5 percent as tea, and slightly less than 2 percent as chocolate, with the remainder coming from medications. The variety of amounts and sources of caffeine consumed confounds the ability to determine risk and to make risk management decisions on the use of caffeine for maintenance and enhancement of cognitive performance in military operations. Thus, the military requested the CMNR's assistance in the decision-making process. The request for this review of caffeine's effects on mental performance and its application to military operations originated with Army scientists from the U.S. Army Research Institute of Environmental Medicine and USAMRMC. In October 1998, a subgroup of the CMNR participated in a series of conference calls with USAMRMC and CMNR staff to identify the key areas that should be reviewed and to solicit suggestions for the names of scientists who were active in the research fields of interest.

On February 2–3, 1999, the CMNR convened a workshop in response to a request from Army representatives to provide information on the safety, efficacy, and appropriate doses and formulations of caffeine for transition to field application during military operations. The purpose of the workshop was twofold: first, to evaluate the relevant caffeine research completed since the 1992 CMNR workshop "Food Components to Enhance Performance", particularly research conducted by the military on the ability of caffeine to counteract mental task performance deficits engendered by sleep deprivation, and, second, to review military research on the pharmacokinetics and effectiveness of caffeine-supplemented food bars versus caffeinated chewing gum, and assist the Department of Defense (DOD) in the transition of this research to military application.

The USAMRMC provided specific information and questions for the committee's response. These are included in the later section, Response to Military Questions.

METHODS

One purpose of the study was to organize a workshop to review the scientific data on the efficacy of caffeine in maintaining physical and cognitive performance in military operations, caffeine safety, appropriate formulations for administration during military operations, and to identify any ethical or other considerations. Another purpose was to review the effectiveness of caffeine compared to other compounds that have central nervous system-stimulating effects.

The research presented in this report addresses these issues. Information from the speaker presentations and the published scientific literature, as well as the deliberations of the CMNR, were used in the preparation of this report.

> **NOTE:** It is important to emphasize that the responses to the questions and recommendations in this report are specific to military operations and are not necessarily applicable to the needs of the civilian population. Mental alertness and vigilance in situations of sleep deprivation may be necessary during military operations in order to achieve mission objectives. In the civilian environment, taking large doses of caffeine to offset lack of sleep, especially in situations where public safety and health could potentially be compromised, cannot be justified.

CAFFEINE USE

Caffeine (1,3,7-trimethylxanthine) and the related methylxanthines theobromine (3,7-dimethylxanthine) and theophylline (1,3-dimethylxanthine) are alkaloid compounds widely distributed in plants throughout the world. More than 60 different plant species containing caffeine have been identified. The primary sources of these compounds are coffee (*Caffea arabica*), kola nuts (*Cola acuminata*), tea (*Thea sinensis*), and chocolate (*Cocoa* bean).

Caffeine is the most widely consumed psychoactive or central nervous system stimulant in the world. In addition to its natural occurrence in some foods, caffeine is used as a food additive and as a drug or a component of many pharmaceutical preparations. When administered in the amounts commonly found in foods, beverages, and drugs, it has measurable effects on certain types of human performance.

As a food additive, caffeine is generally considered safe based on a long history of use and on extensive research conducted over more than a century throughout the world. However, despite this long history of use, modern epidemiological techniques have raised concerns about associations between continued use of high levels of caffeine and long-term health.

Amounts of caffeine in commonly used beverages and other products vary a great deal (Table S-1) from as low as 2 mg/8 oz of chocolate milk, to as much as 300 mg/6 oz of strong espresso coffee.

Caffeine intakes in the United States have been estimated based on the available product usage and food consumption data. Mean per capita caffeine intake for all U.S. adults was approximately 3 mg/kg body weight (BW) (equivalent to 180–210 mg for a 60–70-kg person). Mean daily intake for adult consumers of caffeine products was 4 mg/kg BW, and for the ninetieth percentile of caffeine users, intakes approximated 5–7 mg/kg BW.

CAFFEINE METABOLISM

Pharmacology

Caffeine is rapidly and completely absorbed in humans, with 99 percent being absorbed within 45 minutes of ingestion. Peak plasma concentrations occur between 15 and 120 minutes after oral ingestion, and may be influenced by route of administration, the form of administration, or other components of the diet. Once caffeine is absorbed, it is distributed rapidly throughout body water. However, caffeine is also sufficiently lipophilic to pass through all biological membranes and readily crosses the blood–brain barrier. The mean half-life of caffeine in plasma of healthy individuals is about 5 hours, although its half-life may range between 1.5 and 9.5 hours. This wide variation in reported half-life may

TABLE S-1 Caffeine Content of Some Common U.S. Food Products

Item	Average (mg)	Range (mg)
Coffee (5-oz cup)[a]		
Brewed, drip method	120	90–150
Percolated	90	64–124
Instant	75	30–120
Decaffeinated	3	1–5
Espresso (6-oz cup)	240	180–300
Teas (loose or bags, 5-oz cup)[a]		
1-minute brew	21	9–33
3-minute brew	33	20–46
Tea products		
Instant (5-oz cup)	20	12–28
Iced (12-oz glass)	29	22–36
Carbonated beverages	24	20–40
Colas and pepper drinks (12 oz)		
National brands, packaged	42	36–48
National brands, fountain	39	32–48
Store brands, packaged	18	5–29
Citrus drinks (12 oz)		
National brands, packaged	52	43–56
Store brands, packaged	38	26–52
Chocolate products		
Cocoa beverage (8 oz)	6	3–32
Chocolate milk beverage (8 oz)	5	2–7
Milk chocolate (1 oz)	6	1–15
Dark chocolate, semisweet (1 oz)	20	5–35
Baker's chocolate (1 oz)	35	35
Chocolate-flavored syrup (1 oz)	4	4

[a] Note these caffeine amounts are based on a 5-oz cup of beverage. Servings today are more likely to be 8 or 12 oz and caffeine intake should be calculated accordingly.
SOURCE: Adapted from FDA (1980a); Grand and Bell (1997); IFT (1983); Lieberman (1992).

be due to individual variation in excretion rates, or whether the individual smokes (decreases half-life) or uses oral contraceptives (increases half-life).

The pharmacological effects of caffeine (similar to those of other methylxanthines) include mild stimulation and wakefulness, ability to sustain intellectual activity, and decreased reaction times. The fatal acute oral dose of caffeine in humans is estimated to be between 10 and 14 g (150–200 mg/kg). Ingestion of caffeine in doses up to 10 g has caused convulsions and vomiting, with complete recovery in 6 hours. Side effects have also been observed in humans at caffeine intakes of 1 g (15 mg/kg), progressing from mild effects including restlessness, nervousness, and irritability, to more serious effects such as delirium, emesis, neuromuscular tremors, and convulsions.

Physiology

Physiological effects of caffeine include cardiovascular, respiratory, renal, and smooth muscle effects, as well as effects on mood, memory, alertness, and physical and cognitive performance. Caffeine's effect on cognitive function appears to be mediated via several mechanisms: the antagonism of adenosine receptors, the inhibition of phosphodiesterases, the release of calcium from intracellular stores, and antagonism of benzodiazepine receptors. Caffeine's action in blocking adenosine receptors and inhibiting phosphodiesterase appears to be the most important mechanism of action with respect to physiological and behavioral effects.

RESPONSE TO MILITARY QUESTIONS

1. Efficacy: Does CMNR stand by its earlier recommendation that there are sufficient data to recommend a caffeine product to enhance performance? What are the specific indications for use and contraindications for use?

Military personnel face many situations in which extended wakefulness may be required including sentry duty, deployment-related activities, air transportation during emergencies, radar and sonar monitoring, submarine duty, and combat. As part of their duties in these situations, individuals may have to perform complex cognitive tasks. The performance of these tasks is compromised during periods of extended wakefulness.

Caffeine has been shown to induce a variety of positive effects that have contributed to its extensive use worldwide. Caffeine use has been associated with enhanced physical performance, increased alertness, and a countermeasure to the effects of sleep deprivation. Extensive research has been done on each of these effects.

Caffeine use is associated with a reproducible increase in endurance time in physical activities of moderate intensity and long duration with doses of 2–9 mg/kg, in both naive and habituated, trained and untrained test subjects. High-altitude exposure may augment the positive effects of caffeine on endurance performance. Exercise performance is dramatically reduced by altitude exposure, and maximal effort may be diminished by as much as 25 percent. Ingestion of caffeine (4 mg/kg) increased the time to exhaustion at 4,300 m, but not at sea level. This effect was present even after 2 weeks of acclimatization.

Although there is some debate about whether caffeine enhances cognitive performance or simply restores degraded psychomotor performance in rested individuals, a number of studies have demonstrated that caffeine enhances cognitive performance independent of its ability to reverse symptoms of withdrawal and sleep deprivation. Caffeine enhanced accuracy and reduced reaction time on auditory and visual vigilance tasks in a dose-related manner. Moreover, caffeine significantly increased self-reports of vigor and decreased reports of fatigue, depression, and hostility on the Profile of Moods Scale. In a simulated military situation involving a tedious task that required sustained attention for proficient performance (i.e., sentry duty), caffeine eliminated the vigilance decrement that occurred with increasing time on duty, reduced subjective reports of tiredness, and did not impair rifle firing accuracy. Caffeine also increased the number of correct target identifications in both males and females.

Conclusions

Although there is considerable variation in both the doses tested and subjects' responses to the effects of caffeine on cognitive function, overall research shows that caffeine in the range of 100 to 600 mg is effective in increasing the speed of reaction time without affecting accuracy and in improving performance on visual and audio vigilance tasks. A number of studies have also reported improved performance on long-term memory recall, but not short-term word recall. These enhancing effects of caffeine on cognitive performance are most pronounced when functions are impaired or suboptimal (e.g., as a result of sleep deprivation).

Furthermore, caffeine in amounts ranging from 200 to 600 mg/d enhances endurance performance in a variety of activities. Limited research has shown caffeine to be especially useful in restoring decrements in physical performance that occur at high altitudes. Food and fluid intake must be monitored carefully when caffeine is used for this purpose, since they are frequently suboptimal in operational situations, especially in extremes of hot and cold environments and at altitude.

Recommendations

Caffeine in doses of 100–600 mg may be used to maintain cognitive performance, particularly in situations of sleep deprivation. Specifically it can be used in maintaining speed of reactions and visual and auditory vigilance, which in military operations could be a life or death situation.

A similar dose range (200–600 mg) of caffeine is also effective in enhancing physical endurance and may be especially useful in restoring some of the physical endurance lost at high altitude.

2. **Safety: What are the medical risks to individuals associated with ready availability of caffeine, including acute health risks, long-term health risks, potential interaction with other drugs or factors specific to military operations, and potential problems of habituation of use?**

The effect of caffeine on various aspects of health has been and continues to be an active area of scientific research, in spite of the fact that caffeine has been used by people around the world for more than 1,000 years without apparent ill effects. Extensive research has been done to evaluate the impact of caffeine consumption on the incidence of cardiovascular disease, reproduction and pregnancy outcomes, fluid homeostasis, and osteoporosis. It has been shown that ingestion of very high doses of caffeine can produce undesirable effects on mental function. Additionally, caffeine use has been associated with physical dependence, which may be reflected in performance decrements during withdrawal under some circumstances.

Potential Health Risks

Hypertension

Results summarized in recent reviews suggest that caffeine-naive individuals experience a small increase in blood pressure after acute dosing with caffeine. During chronic administration of caffeine, tolerance appears to develop, and chronic, long-lasting changes in blood pressure are usually not seen in individuals who consume caffeine routinely.

A recent critical review of 30 years of research on the blood pressure effects of coffee and caffeine concluded that the acute pressor effects of caffeine are well documented, but that at present there is no clear epidemiological evidence that caffeine consumption is causally related to hypertension. One potential risk should be noted, however. A number of studies have demonstrated that caffeine consumption produces a transient elevation in blood pressure and that this occurs regardless of whether or not the individual is a habitual user of caffeine. Thus, high caffeine intake may be an additional risk factor for hypertension at the individual level due to long-lasting stress or genetic susceptibility to hypertension.

Heart Disease

In general, controlled clinical attempts to demonstrate effects of caffeine on increasing heart rate or inducing arrhythmia have been unsuccessful. A meta-analysis of 11 prospective, longitudinal cohort studies showed no increased risk of coronary heart disease associated with consumption of up to 6 cups of coffee per day. Thus, increased risk of cardiovascular problems resulting from the use of caffeine supplements by the military would not appear to be of major concern.

Reproduction

Caffeine consumption has been suggested as the cause of numerous negative reproductive outcomes, from shortened menstrual cycles to reduced conception, delayed implantation, spontaneous abortion, premature birth, low infant birthweight, and congenital malformations. As with most other aspects of caffeine consumption, there is a paucity of reliable data concerning the effects of caffeine on reproductive processes.

Recent reviews of human studies suggest that some of the initial reported associations between caffeine and reduced fertility, teratogenicity, and other fetal and maternal effects in humans may be explained by confounding factors such as associated cigarette smoking, alcohol consumption, reporting inaccuracies, and other methodological errors. A recent, well-controlled study using serum paraxanthine levels to quantitate caffeine exposure demonstrated that women who had spontaneous abortions also had significantly higher serum paraxanthine. However, the odds ratio for spontaneous abortion was not significantly increased except in subjects with extremely high paraxanthine levels (> 1,845 ng/mL). The authors concluded that moderate consumption of caffeine was not likely to increase the risk of spontaneous abortion.

Osteoporosis

Caffeine consumption has also been proposed as a risk factor for osteoporosis. In the large number of studies that have been conducted, there appears to be no consistent trend linking caffeine consumption and negative effects on bone mineral density or incidence of fracture. Early studies also indicated a significant effect on acute calcium diuresis; however, subsequent work indicated that this acute phase of excretion was accompanied by a later decrease in excretion of calcium in the urine. Later studies found either no significant effect of caffeine on calcium balance or negative balance only in subjects consuming less than half of the currently recommended intake of calcium.

Fluid Homeostasis

Caffeine is a diuretic and has been found to increase urinary excretion within 1 hour of treatment. Significant increases have been observed in 3-hour urine output as well as in 24-hour urine output as a result of caffeine consumption in amounts of 250 to 642 mg. Currently, data are inconsistent with respect to whether caffeine creates a total body water deficit. The deficit may depend on the amount of caffeine consumed, the individual's history of caffeine use, and the total solute load of any accompanying food or beverage. However, the risk of water deficit may be increased when caffeine is used in situations already known to put personnel at risk of dehydration such as in hot or desert environments (IOM, 1993) or in cold environments (IOM, 1996).

Behavioral Effects

One potential risk of high doses of caffeine, which needs further substantiation, is a dose-related decrement in mental functioning. A number of researchers have found that high doses of caffeine can adversely affect mental performance. Although a relatively low dose of caffeine (250 mg) produced favorable subjective effects (e.g., elation and pleasantness) and enhanced performance on cognitive tasks in healthy volunteers, higher doses (500 mg) led to less favorable subjective reports (e.g., tension, nervousness, anxiety, restlessness) and less improvement in cognitive performance than placebo. Negative effects may be more pronounced in nonusers than in regular users of caffeine. Excessive intake of caffeine (caffeinism) may be mistaken for anxiety disorder.

Physical Dependence and Withdrawal

The use of caffeine by humans is generally not associated with abuse or addiction. Tolerance develops to some of the effects of caffeine when caffeine-containing beverages are consumed regularly. Withdrawal symptoms often occur with the abrupt removal of caffeine from the diet. The frequency of occurrence of withdrawal varies anywhere from 4 to 100 percent. The symptoms of cessation, when they do occur, are not long-lasting and are generally mild. These include headaches, drowsiness, irritability, fatigue, low vigor, and flu-like symptoms. This withdrawal phenomenon could conceivably lead to decrements in performance during military operations.

Caffeine and Stress

Among the variables that may contribute to differences in caffeine sensitivity are baseline levels of stressor exposure and genetically mediated stress reactivity. Stress may include physical stressors (e.g., exercise) physiological stressors (e.g., heat stress, infection, sleep deprivation), or psychological stressors. After stressor exposures, stress-responsive neurohormonal and neurotransmitter systems are activated. Caffeine alters the degree of responsiveness of these stress-responsive systems to stressful stimuli. The degree to which responsiveness is altered varies according to previous caffeine consumption (habitual users versus nonusers).

Conclusions

The acute pressor effects of caffeine are well documented, but at present there is no clear epidemiological evidence that caffeine consumption is causally related to hypertension. However, high caffeine intake may be an additional risk factor for hypertension at the individual level. In borderline-hypertensive men, the use of caffeine in situations of behavioral stress may elevate blood pressure to a clinically meaningful degree.

Since military scenarios in which use of caffeine supplements might be desirable would frequently occur when personnel are also under acute mental and/or physical stress, this could be a concern to personnel with family histories of hypertension.

Increased risk of cardiovascular problems resulting from the use of caffeine supplements by the military would not appear to be of major concern.

Results of studies of the effects of caffeine on reproduction have been very mixed, and many studies showing increased reproductive problems have been confounded with other life-style factors, particularly smoking. The most convincing evidence relates to caffeine and the small increased risk of spontaneous abortion. However, since this requires caffeine consumption during the first trimester of pregnancy, it is unlikely to be a major concern for sustained military operations.

The preponderance of research on caffeine and osteoporosis has found no effect. Although caffeine can increase calcium diuresis, this is compensated by lower than normal calcium excretion later. The use of caffeine in this case is less of a concern than is low calcium intake.

Caffeine may increase risk of dehydration which may be an issue for military personnel in operational environments where dehydration may already be a concern, such as desert environments, or where thirst mechanisms are inadequate such as in cold or high-altitude environments.

High doses of caffeine (> 600 mg) can cause decrements in cognitive function. Caffeine can also potentiate the effects of stress.

Recommendations

Use of caffeine under conditions of sustained military operations would not appear to pose any serious, irreversible acute or chronic health risks for military personnel in situations where increased doses might be recommended.

Caffeine use in sustained operations in hot or cold environments or at high altitudes may increase the risk of dehydration, so fluid and food intake of personnel should be closely monitored in these situations.

Female military personnel should be advised of the potential for a small increased risk of spontaneous abortion in the first trimester of pregnancy.

3. Dose and Warning Labels: What dose level should be recommended to habituated caffeine users and to nonusers? What warnings should be provided on such a product in the context of ethical, religious, and potential caffeine habituation concerns?

The effective dose of caffeine will vary from individual to individual, depending on a variety of factors including time of day, usual caffeine intake, and whether the individual is rested or fatigued. Levels of caffeine in the range of 100 to 400 mg have consistently demonstrated reductions in reaction time and enhanced performance on vigilance tests without adverse effects. In some studies with rested subjects, levels of caffeine in excess of 500 mg in a single dose have shown negative effects on mood and behavior (this may be more likely in those who do not normally consume caffeine). The levels of caffeine that have consistently enhanced physical endurance in humans range from about 200 to 600 mg.

In sleep-deprived individuals, similar to those engaging in sustained operations, a range of 100 to 600 mg of caffeine appears to improve performance (e.g., vigilance, mood, higher cognitive functions) with few acute adverse behavioral effects.

Important ethical considerations for requiring the use of caffeine during sustained operations include: providing personnel with adequate information on use of the product, development of a product that would allow individual control of the dosage, and provision of information on potential negative effects that may be experienced if higher than recommended amounts are consumed.

Individuals who are regular moderate to heavy users of caffeine may experience headaches, fatigue, and other adverse effects if denied access to caffeine in anticipation of the later need to use a supplement.

Conclusions

A caffeine dose of 100–600 mg can be expected to improve vigilance and enhance cognitive performance. A delivery mechanism that provides caffeine in 100-mg increments could be used to allow individuals of smaller body size, non-habituated caffeine users, and those with a heightened sensitivity to caffeine to use the product.

The recommended dosing interval should take into consideration that too-frequent dosing might produce a build-up of caffeine and its metabolite paraxanthine sufficient to precipitate negative effects, or inhibit sleep onset in some individuals when sleep is desired.

The committee concludes that there is no specific need to include warning or cautionary statements on the product labels, and the dosage recommended is well within the range of caffeine consumption in the general population.

Recommendations

A caffeine delivery vehicle that provides caffeine in 100-mg increments with a total content not exceeding approximately 600 mg would appear to be the most appropriate dose for use in sustained military operations. No differential dosing is recommended for habitual and first-time caffeine users. However, a single dose should not exceed 600 mg, and 400 mg may be adequate for rested individuals performing sustained vigilance tasks.

Since the average half-life of caffeine in the blood of adult men given 280 mg (4 mg/kg BW) is between 2.5 and 4.5 hours, a dosing interval of no less than 3–4 hours is suggested.

Any product that is used as a vehicle for providing caffeine to military personnel should be prominently labeled, including a statement on the principal display panel that the product contains added caffeine and should be used only to maintain performance when involved in sustained operations.

The label should also indicate the amount of caffeine per unit of product (or per serving) and instructions for use. This information is vital for commanders to make decisions about directives for use and for personnel to adapt consumption to their individual needs.

An in-depth training program on the benefits, directions for use, and potential side effects of caffeine should be designed for command personnel. Military personnel should be given adequate training to ensure the benefits of caffeine supplementation and avoid any potential side effects. Such training should include the use of caffeine during periods of sleep deprivation and altered work–rest cycles in nonoperational situations.

Military personnel who are habitual consumers of caffeine should not be restricted from caffeine use in preparation for the need of a caffeine supplement.

4. Alternatives: Are there practical alternatives to caffeine that would better serve the intended purpose of enhancing or maintaining performance in fatigued service members?

Sleep is the most effective means of reconstituting the decrements in cognitive functioning brought on by sleep deprivation. Thus, in situations where it is feasible, sleep should be promoted. There is a dose effect for the restorative effects of sleep duration on cognitive performance. Any amount of sleep from as little as a 15-minute nap can restore some degree of function, although the longer the sleep episode, the greater the amount of cognitive function restored.

Alternatives

Combination of Caffeine and Naps

The most effective nonprescription alternative to caffeine administration alone is a combination of caffeine and naps. In a series of studies, the combination of a short nap and caffeine significantly decreased driving impairment, subjective sleepiness, and drowsiness as measured by electroencephalogram activity. The combination of a nap and caffeine also increased alertness during long periods of sleep deprivation as compared to either caffeine or nap treatments independently.

Amphetamine

Amphetamine has been found to "improve subjective feelings of fatigue, confusion, and depression while increasing feelings of vigor". Amphetamine is, however, a controlled substance and its use would require an individual medical evaluation to determine risk factors and health status before a prescription could be issued. It is possible that with appropriate supervision and control, amphetamine could provide benefits to individuals with unique skills and whose performance is critical to the safety of complex military hardware and personnel.

The potential for abuse of amphetamine is considerable. Appropriate monitoring of its dispensation and use may add unnecessary burdens to personnel involved in the intense and demanding tasks that are directly related to the success of sustained operations (SUSOPS). Although amphetamine (20 mg) was more effective than caffeine at 300 mg in reversing the negative effects on alertness during sleep deprivation, it had deleterious effects on recovery sleep, which also may be important in the ultimate success of demanding and constantly changing SUSOPS. Therefore, considerable caution is warranted, and use of this stimulant should be restricted to circumstances when such measures are considered essential to the success of highly sensitive operations.

Modafinil

Modafinil is a controlled wakefulness-promoting drug developed to counteract excessive daytime sleepiness (EDS) in narcolepsy. This drug appears to be useful in reducing EDS without affecting voluntary naps or nocturnal sleep initiation. These properties suggest that this compound may be useful in extending high levels of vigilance in SUSOPS. The limited research to date on the effects of modafinil in simulated military situations indicates potential for this drug.

Conclusions

Providing the opportunity and environment for adequate sleep would be ideal, but obviously impractical, for continuous military operations. Combining naps with judicious caffeine use may be the best remedy for sleep deprivation-induced decrements in cognitive function in military situations where adequate sleep cannot be obtained. When naps are not an option, caffeine alone could be used.

The use of amphetamine is superior to caffeine in offsetting decrements in cognitive performance; however, the risks outweigh the benefits for most situations. It is a controlled substance, has a high abuse potential, and interferes with recovery sleep. In addition, it is assumed that the majority of combat personnel would not have previous experience with the drug.

The drug modafinil, developed as a treatment for narcolepsy, shows considerable promise. It appears to be as effective as amphetamine in offsetting performance degradation, does not interfere with initiation of recovery sleep, is not an appetite suppressant, and appears to have a much lower abuse potential.

Recommendations

It is recommended that the military have in place a doctrine related to the importance of sleep prior to extended missions, the importance of naps whenever possible during operations, and the timing of naps for maximum effectiveness.

Of the psychostimulant compounds that have been thoroughly tested, caffeine would be the compound of choice. Many personnel would have personal experience with the compound, it is not a restricted substance, it does not interfere with recovery sleep following periods of sleep deprivation, and it has very low abuse potential.

Additional research should be conducted on the drug modafinil to further explore its potential for sustaining cognitive performance during military operations.

5. **Formulation: (a) Does the inclusion of other components (e.g., glucose) improve the beneficial effects of caffeine in sustained operations, as previously suggested by the committee? (b) Is there a better approach to caffeine delivery than the nutrient bar (HOOAH) currently produced for the military?**

The evidence of the utility of adding glucose or other components to caffeine to further enhance performance is unclear. Caffeine enhances the availability of free fatty acids and decreases glycogenolysis, whereas carbohydrate increases the availability, and presumably the use, of glucose.

There may be nutritional reasons (e.g., provision of food energy, nutrients, or fluid) for including caffeine in a food or beverage form. Various approaches to caffeine delivery for SUSOPS were considered, including a food/energy bar, caffeinated chewing gum, tablets (both sustained release and regular), and beverages. There is good evidence that caffeine consumed as a liquid is absorbed rapidly and completely from the gut, with virtually all (99 percent) of the administered dose absorbed in about 45 minutes. However, evidence on absorption of caffeine from a food matrix, such as energy bars, was not available.

A caffeine delivery vehicle that is most appropriate in one setting may not be so in another. Caffeine in a food matrix or beverage may be advantageous when it is important to deliver nutrients, fluid, or other food constituents simultaneously. Chewing gums are more appropriate if rapid absorption and action are needed, or weight or bulk is a concern. Caffeine in a fluid matrix or gel may be more appropriate when dehydration is a concern.

Conclusions

Although evidence of a potentiating effect of carbohydrates on caffeine effectiveness is equivocal, there are other reasons to consider providing supplemental nutrients along with the caffeine. Inadequate food and fluid intake is a common problem during military operations.

The use of a caffeinated chewing gum would appear to provide the most rapid absorption. Environmental circumstances and individual characteristics may make one caffeine delivery vehicle appropriate in some circumstances and inappropriate in others.

Recommendations

Definitive research is needed regarding the combined effects of caffeine and carbohydrate on performance since data currently available are inconclusive.

If a food bar or some other solid food matrix is used, the rapidity and extent of caffeine absorption and action must be evaluated.

Under certain circumstances, such as heat stress or desert operations, chewing gums may offer practical operational advantages over a food/energy bar. Thus, two delivery vehicles should be considered. Based on the DOD preference to provide needed supplements to personnel in food form rather than in pill form, a caffeinated chewing gum or a caffeine-supplemented food/energy bar would be suitable delivery vehicles.

1

Basic Concepts

MILITARY INTEREST IN CAFFEINE

Optimal job performance without compromising the health and well-being of the worker is the goal of employers regardless of the field of endeavor. Intermittent or prolonged physiological and psychological stressors that employees bring to the workplace have an impact not only on their own performance but also on those with whom they work and interact. The internal stressors an individual brings to his or her job are compounded by the day-to-day physical and mental stressors of the job itself. Military personnel in combat settings endure highly unpredictable timing and types of stressors as well as situations that require continuing vigilance for long periods of time.

The U.S. military's concerns about the individual war fighter's ability to avoid performance degradation and the need to enhance mental capabilities in highly stressful situations have led to an interest in devising military ration components that could enhance physical and cognitive performance.

Previous Committee on Military Nutrition Research Recommendations

In 1992 the Committee on Military Nutrition Research (CMNR) was asked by the U.S. Army Medical Research and Materiel Command to evaluate the potential of selected amino acids, carbohydrates, structured lipids, choline, carnitine, and caffeine to enhance performance. The committee was asked to address two questions: first, whether the use of diet components or supplements to enhance physical and mental performance in "normal" healthy, young adult soldiers was a fruitful approach and, second, which food components, if any, would be the best candidates for enhancing military mental and physical performance. In response to this request the committee held a workshop, reviewed the scientific literature, and published the report, *Food Components to Enhance Performance* (IOM, 1994), in which it recommended continued research on the mechanisms of the effects of caffeine on cognitive performance, mood, and alertness. It was noted that particular attention should be paid to maximizing positive effects when performance is already degraded.

Specifically, the committee recommended:

> Caffeine definitely should be considered in developing performance-enhancing rations or ration components. Caffeine is safe as a component of food at doses required to overcome sleep deprivation and has already been included in diets of military personnel via coffee and many soft drinks. Since many soldiers may not normally drink coffee, a mechanism for including caffeine in another ration component that can be selectively used when the situation requires should be evaluated. It appears that doses of 300–600 mg/70 kg person will achieve the desired stimulus in those nonhabituated to caffeine; additional research needs to be conducted to determine the effects of this level of caffeine in those with higher habitual intakes. (IOM, 1994, p. 50)

The Current Situation

Changes in military operations over the last 50 years have forced continued assessment and adoption of technologies that will sustain or enhance physical and cognitive performance of the individual service member. This urgency in maintaining and enhancing performance is fostered by increased reliance on the individual's cognitive skills in the operation and maintenance of complex military equipment in an ever-increasing variety of environmental conditions. Today's military relies heavily on the use of computer-controlled systems that require highly trained and alert operators. In addition, there is greater reliance on rapid mobility to enable deployment at any time to achieve the nation's military objectives. The urgency of maintaining and enhancing performance is also driven by constant pressure, due to personnel reductions, to have the individual perform for longer periods of time with less sleep, shorter transition times, less recovery time between missions, and less reliance on traditional logistical support.

These scenarios can have severe impacts on the individual's level of fatigue, alertness, response time, mood, judgment, reliability in decision making, and other cognitive skills. Increased likelihood of decrements in cognitive function is coupled with greater dependence on each individual in accomplishment of the mission. Both of these factors have a profound impact on the success or failure of a military operation.

In its effort to sustain and enhance the performance of personnel, the military's emphasis should be placed on providing adequate levels of nutrients, water, life support equipment, clothing, and, to the extent possible, sleeping regimens, appropriate rest areas, and work patterns. After these efforts have been put in place, the potential use of dietary supplements and selected pharmaceuticals is an appropriate consideration.

HISTORY OF CAFFEINE USE

In addition to its natural occurrence in some foods, caffeine is used as a food additive and as a drug or a component of many pharmaceutical preparations. It is the most widely consumed psychoactive or central nervous system (CNS) stimulant in the world (Curatolo and Robertson, 1983). When administered in the doses commonly found in beverages and drugs, it has measurable effects on certain types of human performance. It is readily available to both the civilian and the military populations as a beverage (coffee, tea, maté), food (cocoa products), food additive (soft drinks, bottled water), and pharmaceutical (over-the-counter pain and weight-loss medications, numerous prescription drugs). No other substance has this combination of uses.

As a food additive caffeine is generally considered safe based on its long history of use and on extensive research conducted throughout the world for more than a century. However, despite this long history of use, modern epidemiological techniques have raised concerns about associations between continued use of high levels of caffeine and long-term health.

Caffeine (1,3,7-trimethylxanthine) and the related methylxanthines, theobromine (3,7-dimethylxanthine) and theophylline (1,3-dimethylxanthine), are widely distributed in plants throughout the world. More than 60 different plant species containing caffeine have been identified, and history suggests that it may have been consumed, in one form or another, as far back as the Paleolithic period (Barone and Roberts, 1996). The primary sources of these compounds are coffee (*Caffea arabica*), kola nuts (*Cola acuminata*), tea (*Thea sinensis*), and chocolate (*Cocoa* bean). Although the actual discoverer of caffeine as a stimulant is unknown, legend has it that it was first discovered in Ethiopia in the third century AD when a shepherd noticed that his goats became very frisky and agitated after eating coffee berries or "beans". The shepherd tried chewing some of the berries and noted their stimulant properties. An abbot at a nearby monastery brewed the beans in hot water and found that the beverage helped him to stay awake during long nights of prayer. Cultivation of the coffee plant may have begun as early as the sixth century AD, probably in Ethiopia. Elsewhere in Africa, coffee berries were crushed and mixed with fat to serve as a food to stimulate warriors in battle. By approximately 1000 AD, coffee reached Yemen, where the beverage became very popular and drinking it a social ritual among Muslims. From there it spread to Europe and the Americas. All stable indigenous cultures having access to caffeine-containing plants have developed drinks or foods containing these stimulant products. The earliest recorded use of caffeine-containing beverages dates back to the Tang Dynasty of China (618–907 AD) where tea was a popular drink believed to prolong life.

Caffeine Content of Common Food Sources

The amount of caffeine in commonly consumed beverages and other products varies a great deal (Table 1-1), from as little as 5 mg/8 oz of chocolate milk, to as much as 300 mg/6 oz of strong espresso coffee. Since early times the adverse effects of very large doses of caffeine, especially in those who are not used to the product, have been noted. The reported signs and symptoms include nervousness, anxiety, insomnia, irregular heartbeats, excess stomach acid, and heartburn (Duke, 1988).

Caffeine Intake of Adults

Based on the available product usage data and food consumption data, Barone and Roberts (1996) estimated caffeine intakes in the United States, United Kingdom, Denmark, and Australia. The per capita daily caffeine intake for all U.S. adults was approximately 3 mg/kg body weight (BW) (for a 60–70-kg person). For adults who actually consumed caffeine products, mean daily intake was 4 mg/kg BW, and for the ninetieth percentile of caffeine users, intakes approximated 5–7 mg/kg BW.

Caffeine intake was higher in the United Kingdom, with per capita daily consumption being 4 mg/kg BW and 7.5 mg/kg BW for the ninetieth percentile of caffeine users. Consumption was highest in Denmark: 7.0 mg/kg BW for all adults and 14.9 mg/kg BW for the ninetieth percentile of caffeine users.

THE COMMITTEE'S TASK

Surveys indicate that more than 90 percent of the military population consumes caffeine at some level on a daily basis. A small-sample survey reported by Lieberman (1999) indicated that mean caffeine intake among military personnel was 340 mg/d. The majority of those sampled consumed 200 mg/d or less; however, consumption levels were highly variable and thus physiological effects cannot be generalized. Typically, older personnel consumed more caffeine than younger ones, and males consumed slightly more than females. The majority of caffeine (about 70 percent) was consumed as coffee, 23 percent as soda, 5 percent as tea, and slightly less than 2 percent as chocolate, with the remainder coming from medications. These factors make it difficult to determine risk and to make risk management decisions on the use of caffeine for maintenance and enhancement of cognitive performance in military operations.

TABLE 1-1 Caffeine Content of Some Common U.S. Food Products

Item	Average (mg)	Range (mg)
Coffee (5-oz cup)[a]		
Brewed, drip method	120	90–150
Percolated	90	64–124
Instant	75	30–120
Decaffeinated	3	1–5
Espresso (6-oz cup)	240	180–300
Teas (loose or bags, 5-oz cup)[a]		
1-minute brew	21	9–33
3-minute brew	33	20–46
Tea products		
Instant (5-oz cup)	20	12–28
Iced (12-oz glass)	29	22–36
Carbonated beverages	24	20–40
Colas and pepper drinks (12 oz)		
National brands, packaged	42	36–48
National brands, fountain	39	32–48
Store brands, packaged	18	5–29
Citrus drinks (12 oz)		
National brands, packaged	52	43–56
Store brands, packaged	38	26–52
Chocolate products		
Cocoa beverage (8 oz)	6	3–32
Chocolate milk beverage (8 oz)	5	2–7
Milk chocolate (1 oz)	6	1–15
Dark chocolate, semisweet (1 oz)	20	5–35
Baker's chocolate (1 oz)	35	35
Chocolate-flavored syrup (1 oz)	4	4

[a] Note these caffeine amounts are based on a 5-oz cup of beverage, servings today are more likely to be 8 or 12 oz and caffeine intake should be calculated accordingly.
SOURCE: Adapted from FDA (1980a); Grand and Bell (1997); IFT (1983); Lieberman (1992).

The military requested the committee's assistance in this decision-making process. The CMNR was requested to evaluate the relevant caffeine research, including all relevant studies performed since the 1992 workshop, and address in a brief report the following proposal and questions to assist the Department of Defense in the transition of research to military application. Specifically, the military provided the following information and questions for the committee's response.

A specific transition opportunity could take the following form: a "HOOAH" food bar (a nutrient-dense energy bar developed by the Army) containing 600 mg of caffeine, scored in 150-mg increments, with labeling that provides specific guidance for use of up to one food bar (600 mg) to offset deficits in cognitive function and situational awareness produced by inadequate restorative sleep and during military operations at night. The label should also contain warnings, especially for infrequent or noncaffeine users, that no more than one scored segment (150 mg) should be used in the first hour and should be discontinued if undesirable changes in hand steadiness, pulse, and respiration occur. This performance-enhancing ration component could be provided separately or as part of operational rations. Alternatives to be considered include coffee, caffeinated soft drinks, modifications of the HOOAH bar dose, caffeinated chewing gum, caffeine pills, amphetamine pills (dexedrine), and sustained-release caffeine. The intent is to provide a pharmacological/dietary supplement strategy to significantly counter performance deficits in special circumstances when doctrinal and behavioral solutions (adherence to appropriate work–rest cycles, naps, etc.) are not possible or break down. The key questions to be addressed:

1. *Efficacy:* Does the committee stand by its earlier recommendation that there are sufficient data to recommend a caffeine product to enhance performance, and what are the specific indications for use (e.g., vigilance activities following inadequate sleep) and contraindications for use (e.g., tasks involving fine motor coordination)?

2. *Safety:* What are the medical risks to individuals associated with ready availability of caffeine, including acute health risks (e.g., cardiac arrhythmia, caffeine psychosis), long-term health risks (e.g., hypertension, hypercholesterolemia), potential interactions with other drugs (e.g., ephedra-containing supplements) or factors specific to military operations (e.g., heat stress, stress reactions), and potential problems of habituation of use (e.g., tolerance, caffeine dependence)?

3. *Dose and warning labels:* What dose level(s) should be recommended to (a) habituated caffeine users and (b) nonhabituated users? What warnings should be provided on such a product in the context of ethical, religious, and potential caffeine habituation concerns?

4. *Alternatives:* Are there practical alternatives to caffeine, which would better serve the intended purpose of enhancing performance in fatigued service members (e.g., amphetamine)?

5. *Formulation:* (a) Does the inclusion of other components (e.g., glucose) improve beneficial effects of caffeine in sustained operations (SUSOPS), as previously suggested by the committee? (b) Is there a better approach to caffeine delivery than the HOOAH bar (e.g., is it better to have more rapid absorption and action using caffeinated chewing gum, longer duration of action using sustained-release caffeine products, or pill or beverage formulations)?

A workshop was organized to review the scientific data on the efficacy of caffeine in maintaining physical and cognitive performance in military operations, its safety, and appropriate formulations for administration during military operations and to identify any ethical or other considerations. Another purpose of this workshop was to compare the effectiveness of caffeine to other pharmaceuticals that have CNS effects.

The research presented at this workshop addressed many of these issues. Information from the speaker presentations and the published scientific literature, as well as the deliberations of the CMNR, were used in the preparation of this report.

> **NOTE:** It is important to emphasize that the responses to the questions and recommendations in this report are specific to military operations and are not necessarily applicable to the needs of the civilian population. In particular, it is recognized that mental alertness and vigilance in situations of sleep deprivation may be necessary during military operations in order to achieve mission objectives. In the civilian environment, taking large doses of caffeine to offset lack of sleep in situations where public safety and health could potentially be compromised, such as in the operation of aircraft, motor vehicles, heavy equipment, delicate life-saving procedures, and the like, is not justified.

2

Pharmacology of Caffeine

As stated in Chapter 1, caffeine is the most widely used central nervous system (CNS) stimulant in the world. It has numerous pharmacological and physiological effects, including cardiovascular, respiratory, renal, and smooth muscle effects, as well as effects on mood, memory, alertness, and physical and cognitive performance. This chapter provides a brief summary of the metabolism and physiological effects of caffeine

Caffeine (1,3,7-trimethylxanthine) is a plant alkaloid with a chemical structure of $C_8H_{10}N_4O_2$ (see Figure 2-1) and a molecular weight of 194.19. In pure form, it is a bitter white powder. Structurally, caffeine (and the other methylxanthines) resembles the purines. The mean half-life of caffeine in plasma of healthy individuals is about 5 hours. However, caffeine's elimination half-life may range between 1.5 and 9.5 hours, while the total plasma clearance rate for caffeine is estimated to be 0.078 L/h/kg (Brachtel and Richter, 1992; Busto et al., 1989). This wide range in the plasma mean half-life of caffeine is due to both innate individual variation, and a variety of physiological and environmental characteristics that influence caffeine metabolism (e.g., pregnancy, obesity, use of oral contraceptives, smoking, altitude). The pharmacological effects of caffeine are similar to those of other methylxanthines (including those found in various teas and chocolates). These effects include mild CNS stimulation and wakefulness, ability to sustain intellectual activity, and decreased reaction times.

The fatal acute oral dose of caffeine in humans is estimated to be 10–14 g (150–200 mg/kg body weight [BW]) (Hodgman, 1998). Ingestion of caffeine in

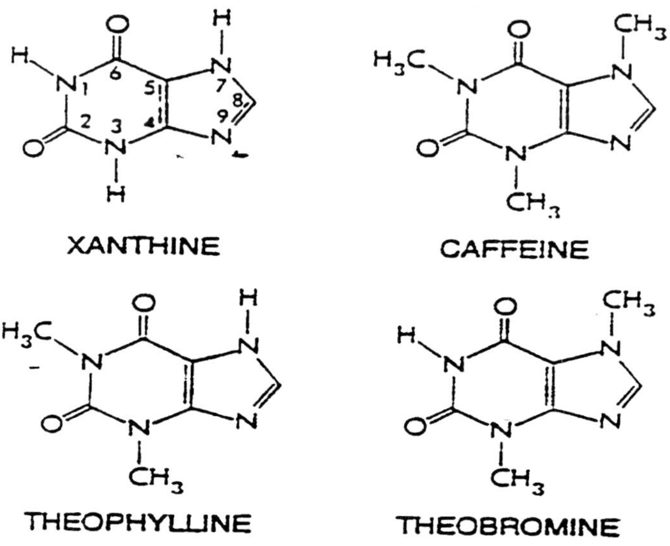

FIGURE 2-1 Chemical structure of methylxanthines.

doses up to 10 g has caused convulsions and vomiting with complete recovery in 6 hours (Dreisbach, 1974). Extreme side effects were observed in humans at caffeine intakes of 1 g (15 mg/kg) (Gilman et al., 1990), including restlessness, nervousness, and irritability, and progressing to delirium, emesis, neuromuscular tremors, and convulsions. Other symptoms included tachycardia and increased respiration.

ABSORPTION, DISTRIBUTION, AND METABOLISM

Caffeine is rapidly and completely absorbed in humans, with 99 percent being absorbed within 45 minutes of ingestion (Bonati et al., 1982; Liguori et al., 1997). When it is consumed in beverages (most commonly coffee, tea, or soft drinks) caffeine is absorbed rapidly from the gastrointestinal tract and distributed throughout body water. More rapid absorption can be achieved by chewing caffeine-containing gum or other preparations that allow absorption through the oral mucosa.

Peak plasma concentrations occur between 15 and 120 minutes after oral ingestion. This wide variation in time may be due to variation in gastric emptying time and the presence of other dietary constituents, such as fiber (Arnaud, 1987). Once caffeine is absorbed, there appears to be no hepatic first-pass effect (i.e., the liver does not appear to remove caffeine as it passes from the gut to the general circulation), as evidenced by the similarity in plasma concentration curves that follow its administration by either the oral or the intravenous route (Arnaud, 1993). Caffeine binds reversibly to plasma proteins, and protein-bound caffeine accounts for about 10 to 30 percent of the total plasma pool. The distribution volume within the body is 0.7 L/kg, a value suggesting that it is hydrophilic and distributes freely into the intracellular tissue water (Arnaud, 1987, 1993). However, caffeine is also sufficiently lipophilic to pass through all biological membranes and readily crosses the blood–brain barrier. Its elimination is by first-order kinetics and is adequately described by a one-compartment open model system (Bonati et al., 1982). In a study of adult men, a dose of 4 mg/kg (280 mg/70 kg human, or about 2–3 cups of coffee) had a caffeine half-life of 2.5–4.5 hours, and was not affected by age (Arnaud, 1988).

Because caffeine is readily reabsorbed by the renal tubules, once it is filtered by the glomeruli only a small percentage is excreted unchanged in the urine. Its limited appearance in urine indicates that caffeine metabolism is the rate-limiting factor in its plasma clearance (Arnaud, 1993). Caffeine metabolism occurs primarily in the liver, catalyzed by hepatic microsomal enzyme systems (Grant et al., 1987). In healthy humans, repeated caffeine ingestion does not alter its absorption or metabolism (George et al., 1986). It is metabolized in the liver to dimethylxanthines, uric acids, di- and trimethylallantoin, and uracil derivatives. In humans 3-ethyl demethylation to paraxanthine is the primary route of metabolism (Arnaud, 1987). This first metabolic step accounts for approximately 75–80 percent of caffeine metabolism and involves cytochrome P4501A2 (Arnaud, 1993). Paraxanthine is the dominant metabolite in humans, rising in plasma to concentrations 10 times those of theophylline or theobromine. Caffeine is cleared more quickly than paraxanthine, so 8 to 10 hours after caffeine ingestion, paraxanthine levels exceed caffeine levels in plasma (Arnaud, 1993).

The fact that the human body converts 70–80 percent of caffeine into paraxanthine with no apparent toxic effects following caffeine doses of 300–500 mg/day suggests that paraxanthine's toxicological potency is low. Formation of paraxanthine and its excretion in the urine appears to be the major pathway for caffeine metabolism (Stavric, 1988).

Hetzler et al. (1990) demonstrated that lipolytic effects of caffeine may be due to the action of paraxanthine rather than caffeine itself. Increasing concentration of plasma-free fatty acids following intravenous administration of caffeine was negatively correlated to plasma caffeine concentrations, and highly positively correlated to plasma paraxanthine concentrations. Paraxanthine has been found to be an equipotent adenosine antagonist to caffeine in vitro. Benowitz et al. (1995) demonstrated that both caffeine and paraxanthine significantly increased diastolic blood pressure, plasma concentrations of epinephrine, and free fatty acids. Plasma levels of caffeine peaked 75 minutes after oral dosing of caffeine, while plasma levels of paraxanthine peaked at 300 minutes after an oral dose of paraxanthine. At doses of 4 mg/kg BW, caffeine and paraxanthine were equipotent. At doses of 2 mg/kg BW, however, caffeine was more potent. Benowitz and colleagues (1995) concluded that after a single dose of caffeine, paraxanthine concentrations are relatively low and probably do not contribute much to the effect of caffeine. However, with long-term exposure to caffeine there is a substantial accumulation of paraxanthine, and thus paraxanthine almost certainly contributes to the pharmacologic activity of caffeine. It would be reasonable to expect then, that with long-term caffeine exposure, paraxanthine would also contribute to development of tolerance to caffeine and withdrawal symptoms.

There is likely to be considerable individual variation in the extent of conversion of caffeine to paraxanthine, and because paraxanthine has pharmacologic activity, the extent of conversion would be a factor in determining individual differences in response to caffeine.

FACTORS AFFECTING CAFFEINE METABOLISM

Caffeine metabolism is increased by smoking, an effect mediated by an acceleration in its demethylation (it also increases xanthine oxidase activity) (Parsons and Neims, 1978). Smoking cessation returns caffeine clearance rates to nonsmoking values (Murphy et al., 1988). A number of studies with rodents have demonstrated an additive effect of caffeine and nicotine on both schedule-controlled behavior and locomotor activity (Lee et al., 1987; Sansone et al., 1994; White, 1988). However, data in humans are scarce. Kerr et al. (1991) found both caffeine and nicotine facilitated memory and motor function in a variety of psychomotor tasks. Though there were differences across tasks, combining caffeine and nicotine did not appear to produce a greater effect than either drug alone. Conversely, nicotine did not decrease the effectiveness of caffeine.

The effects of caffeine on women have been examined in the context of its effects on menstrual function, interactions with oral contraceptives, pregnancy and fetal health, and postmenopausal health. Earlier studies suggested that elimination of caffeine may vary across the menstrual cycle, with elimination being about 25 percent longer in the luteal phase (Balogh et al., 1987). More recent studies, however, indicate no significant effects on caffeine pharmacokinetics across phases of the menstrual cycle in healthy, nonsmoking women who are not using oral contraceptives (Kamimori et al., 1999). Decreased paraxanthine or caffeine metabolic rates in healthy postmenopausal women on estrogen replacement therapy suggest that exogenous estrogen in older women may inhibit caffeine metabolism through the P450 isozyme CYP1A2, an isozyme common to both estrogen and caffeine metabolism (Pollock et al., 1999). Additionally, it is known that oral contraceptive use can double caffeine half-life (Abernethy and Todd, 1985; Patwardhan et al., 1980). The effects of newer oral contraceptives on caffeine half-life have not been studied.

PHYSIOLOGICAL EFFECTS

Caffeine administration affects the functioning of the cardiovascular, respiratory, renal, and nervous systems. Proposed mechanisms of action differ for different physiological effects. Caffeine action is thought to be mediated via several mechanisms: the antagonism of adenosine receptors, the inhibition of phosphodiesterase, the release of calcium from intracellular stores, and antagonism of benzodiazepine receptors (Myers et al., 1999).

Caffeine and Adenosine Receptors

The ability of caffeine to inhibit adenosine receptors appears to be highly important in its effects on behavior and cognitive function. This ability results from the competitive binding of caffeine and paraxanthine to adenosine receptors and is of importance in contributing to CNS effects, especially those involving the neuromodulatory effects of adenosine. Due to the blocking of adenosine inhibitory effects through its receptors, caffeine indirectly affects the release of norepinephrine, dopamine, acetylcholine, serotonin, glutamate, gamma-aminobutyric acid (GABA), and perhaps neuropeptides (Daly et al., 1999).

There are two main classes of adenosine receptor: A_1 and A_2; caffeine and paraxanthine are nonselective antagonists at both, although they are not especially potent antagonists. The caffeine concentrations attained in vivo that cause mild CNS stimulation (5–10 µM) and that are associated with antiasthmatic effects (50 µM), are in the range associated with adenosine receptor blockade (as quantitated by in vitro receptor binding assays) (Daly, 1993).

Caffeine and Phosphodiesterase

Caffeine increases intracellular concentrations of cyclic adenosine monophosphate (cAMP) by inhibiting phosphodiesterase enzymes in skeletal muscle and adipose tissues. These actions promote lipolysis via the activation of hormone-sensitive lipases with the release of free fatty acids and glycerol. The increased availability of these fuels in skeletal muscle acts to spare the consumption of muscle glycogen. Increased cAMP could also lead to an increase in blood catecholamines. However, caffeine is a fairly weak inhibitor of phosphodiesterase enzymes, and the in vivo concentrations at which behavioral effects occur are probably too low to be associated with meaningful phosphodiesterase inhibition (Burg and Werner, 1975; Daly, 1993).

In contrast, phosphodiesterase inhibition may account for caffeine's (and theophylline's) cardiostimulatory and antiasthmatic actions, since nonxanthine phosphodiesterases are cardiac stimulants (Schmitz et al., 1989) and are also effective as bronchiolar and tracheal relaxants. Indeed, in the latter case, the potency correlates with phosphodiesterase inhibition, not with affinity for adenosine receptors (Brackett et al., 1990; Persson et al., 1982; Polson et al., 1985).

Caffeine and Calcium Mobilization

The earliest proposed mechanism of action for caffeine involved the mobilization of intracellular calcium. Certain actions of caffeine in skeletal muscle appear to involve ionic calcium (Ca^{++}). Caffeine in high concentrations (1–10 mM) was found to interfere with the uptake and storage of calcium in the sarcoplasmic reticulum of striated muscle and to increase the translocation of Ca^{++} through the plasma membrane (Nehlig et al., 1992). Caffeine may also increase myofilamental sensitivity to Ca^{++} through its binding to ryanodine receptors in calcium channels of muscle and brain (McPherson et al., 1991).

Although caffeine has been shown to release calcium from intracellular storage pools (sarcoplasmic reticulum) in skeletal and cardiac muscle, the threshold concentration required in vitro to observe this effect (250 μM) is substantially higher than the concentrations required in vivo for cardiac stimulation (50 μM). Hence, this subcellular action of caffeine is probably physiologically irrelevant (though it conceivably could be relevant at toxic concentrations of caffeine) (Daly, 1993).

Caffeine and Benzodiazepine Receptors

Caffeine modifies or antagonizes the effects of benzodiazepines on behavior in both animals and humans (de Angelis et al., 1982; ME Mattila et al., 1992; MJ Mattila et al., 1992). The mechanism for this antagonism was proposed to be the blocking of benzodiazepine receptors by caffeine. Caffeine does have weak antagonistic properties at these receptors. However, this mechanism requires very high concentrations of caffeine (Nehlig et al., 1987; Weir and Hruska, 1983). More recent evidence (Lopez et al., 1989; Nehlig et al., 1992) suggests that the interaction between caffeine and benzodiazepines is mediated through caffeine's effects on adenosine receptors. There is some evidence that caffeine may also be a histamine receptor antagonist (Acquaviva et al., 1986).

General Effects of Caffeine on Physiological Functions

The effects of caffeine on sodium–potassium–adenosine triphosphate pump activity lead to a decrease in plasma potassium concentrations, and affect the depolarization–repolarization process during exercise with potential effects on fine motor coordination.

The effects of caffeine on the heart are primarily stimulatory and are accompanied by increased coronary blood flow. These effects are thought to be mediated not by an action on adenosine receptors (Collis et al., 1984), but instead via phosphodiesterase inhibition. In the lungs caffeine can cause smooth muscle relaxation and bronchial dilatation, possibly accounting for its antiasthmatic effects. However, the relative roles of adenosine receptors and phosphodiesterase as mechanisms of caffeine's antiasthmatic actions remain unresolved (Brackett and Daly, 1991; Ghai et al., 1987; Persson et al., 1982).

The effects of caffeine on the kidney—diuresis, increased blood flow, and rennin secretion—appear to be due to an action of caffeine at adenosine receptors (Spielman and Arend, 1991). Caffeine's behavioral effects appear to be mediated both through adenosine receptors and phosphodiesterase effects and can readily be seen on neurochemically specific neurons. Caffeine's stimulatory action on dopamine, norepinephrine, serotonin, acetylcholine, glutamate, and GABA neurons is hypothesized to result from its ability to block the action of adenosine, which typically inhibits neuronal function. Phosphodiesterase inhibition by xanthines may also account for some stimulatory effects.

Interactions with other nutrients and drugs also characterize certain effects attributed to caffeine. Such interactions include those associated with aspirin, alcohol, nicotine, cocaine, certain other botanicals, and other narcotics (Callahan et al., 1982; Falk and Lau, 1991; Kuribara and Tadokoro, 1992; Parsons and Neims, 1978; White, 1999).

The repeated administration of caffeine does not change its pharmacokinetics, but in many cases development of tolerance does occur. Tolerance is not observed for all effects of the drug, such as fat cell lipolysis (Holtzman et al., 1991), but is seen for certain behavioral actions, such as some of its stimulant properties (increase in locomotor activity in rats) (Finn and Holtzman, 1986). Following the cessation of caffeine use, withdrawal-like symptoms are sometimes seen in humans, such as headache, irritability, nervousness, and a reduction in energy (Griffiths et al., 1986, 1990). The physiological bases for these symptoms are not known. Although the development of withdrawal symptoms might indicate an addictive property, caffeine does not have a convincing profile as an addictive drug.

SUMMARY

Caffeine is rapidly and completely absorbed within an hour following ingestion. It is distributed throughout body water and readily crosses cell membranes including the brain. Its primary mechanisms for stimulatory activity appear to be the blocking of adenosine receptors and inhibition of phosphodiesterases. Caffeine is metabolized and excreted in humans primarily as paraxanthine, which also has pharmacologic activity. With repeated caffeine dosing, paraxanthine may contribute to development of tolerance and withdrawal symptoms. Caffeine clearance rates are affected by both environmental and physiological factors, such as use of oral contraceptives, smoking, and pregnancy. Tolerance to some of caffeine's physiological affects develops with continued use.

3

Efficacy of Caffeine

Caffeine has been shown clinically to induce a variety of positive effects that have contributed to its extensive use worldwide. Caffeine use has been associated with increased alertness and enhanced physical performance, and as a countermeasure to the effects of sleep deprivation. Extensive research has been done on each of these effects of caffeine. A brief summary of research findings on the efficacy of caffeine is presented here.

PHYSICAL PERFORMANCE

Caffeine has been proposed as an ergogenic aid in physical performance. Its use is associated with a reproducible increase in endurance time in activities of moderate intensity and long duration. Caffeine consumed both at rest and during exercise increases a variety of physiological processes (heart rate, respiratory rate, blood pressure), probably through the secretion of epinephrine. Recent research indicates that caffeine may also act by altering pain perception since it has been reported to increase plasma β-endorphins during endurance exercise (Laurent et al., 2000). Typically, the magnitude of the exercise response far exceeds and masks the resting effects of caffeine intake. However, if the intensity of the exercise is low and the caffeine dose is high, the effect of the caffeine may be obvious even during exercise. Caffeine also shifts cellular metabolism, possibly through antagonism of adenosine receptors (Graham et al., 1994). Specifically, caffeine increases lipolysis via activation of hormone-sensitive lipase, decreases glycogenolysis via direct inhibition of glycogen phosphorylase, and increases blood glucose and oxygen consumption (Spriet, 1999). Earlier work indicated this increase in lipolysis may actually be stimulated by the caffeine metabolite, paraxanthine, rather than by caffeine itself (Hetzler et al., 1990). Energy derived from fat during exercise is increased with caffeine ingestion, while the energy derived from carbohydrate is somewhat reduced at the same intensity of exercise (Sasaki et al., 1987). Glycogen utilization is, at least initially, depressed (Erickson et al., 1987; Essig et al., 1980; Spriet et al., 1992). Blood lactate, which usually increases in exercise above 70–75 percent of VO_{2max}, is not affected by caffeine at rest, and may (Flinn et al., 1990; McNaughton, 1986) or may not (Dodd et al., 1991; Gastin et al., 1990) be affected by caffeine during exercise, depending on the intensity of the exercise and the level of caffeine ingested.

Although in today's military there is an increasing reliance on sophisticated computer-controlled systems, special operations and infantry missions will always rely on the physical fitness of the soldier. These operations consist of either prolonged endurance or brief, high-intensity activity. The efficacy of caffeine in promoting physical performance is different for these two kinds of activity.

Four separate reviews (Dodd et al., 1993; Graham et al., 1994; Spriet, 1995; Tarnopolsky, 1994) have concluded consistently that caffeine enhances endurance performance in a variety of activities (i.e., running, cross-country skiing, cycling), with doses from 2 to 9 mg/kg, in naive and habituated, trained and untrained test subjects. The performance effects are seen at intakes that result in urinary caffeine levels below the legal limits stipulated by the International Olympic Committee and are more pronounced in well-trained athletes (Spriet, 1999).

These same reviews concluded that there was little effect of caffeine on activities requiring high power outputs over a short time, such as lifting, carrying, and sprinting. Such activities utilize primarily anaerobic generation of adenosine triphosphate, a process that is probably not affected by caffeine. In contrast, other studies have shown slightly increased power output due to caffeine intake (Anselme et al., 1992; Collomp et al., 1992; Wiles et al., 1992), or increased time to exhaustion in brief (2-minute) supramaximal exercise (Jackman et al., 1996). This suggests a possible direct effect of caffeine on muscle tissue (Green et al., 1990; Lopes et al., 1983; Tarnopolsky et al., 1992).

Response to caffeine ingestion may vary among studies as a consequence of the caffeine habits of participants. As mentioned elsewhere in this report, chronic use of caffeine results in habituation to some of its effects, possibly by up-regulation of adenosine receptors. The epinephrine response to circulating caffeine or methylxanthine by-products may be attenuated as a result (Tarnopolsky et al., 1989; van Soeren et al., 1993). If the epinephrine response is required for the performance-enhancing effects of caffeine to be realized, habitual users may require a higher dose of caffeine to garner the positive results (Spriet et al., 1992). The dose of caffeine required for significant improvements in physical performance ranges from 3 to 9 mg/kg (Graham and Spriet, 1995). It should be noted, as well, that exercise has been shown to counteract the anxiety that may accompany high doses of caffeine. Youngstedt et al. (1998) showed that after ingestion of 800 mg of caffeine, cycling for 60 minutes at 60 percent of VO_{2max} significantly reduced anxiety compared with consumption of this amount of caffeine while at rest.

Carbohydrate–Caffeine Mixtures

The most important theoretical mechanism of action of caffeine in the context of physical performance of the whole organism is a shift in the primary fuel used for exercise. In adipocytes, caffeine promotes lipolysis by increasing cyclic adenosine monophosphate levels, which in turn increase stimulation of hormone-sensitive lipase. The resulting increase in circulating free fatty acids hypothetically spares muscle glycogen. An independent effect of caffeine on muscle glycogenolysis has also been postulated (as discussed in previous section). In addition, carbohydrate has been shown to enhance performance during continuous exercise lasting at least 50–60 minutes (Armstrong and Maresh, 1996). The hypothesis has been put forward that incorporating the lipolytic qualities of caffeine with the carbohydrate utilization-promoting qualities of carbohydrate ingestion might augment the performance effects of both, suggesting that caffeine delivered in a carbohydrate-containing medium may further enhance performance. The following three studies have tested the efficacy of such a mixture.

Wemple et al. (1997), using a carbohydrate and electrolyte drink (3 mL/kg) with and without caffeine (60 mg per dose), evaluated time to exhaustion at 85 percent VO_{2max} after 3 hours of continuous cycling exercise in six trained subjects. Cycling performance was not affected by including caffeine in the carbohydrate-containing fluid. However, caffeine intake in this experiment was extremely low.

Kovacs et al. (1998) added different doses of caffeine (2–4.5 mg/kg) to a carbohydrate–electrolyte solution and examined the effects on substrate metabolism and endurance performance time in 15 trained subjects during a 1-hour time trial. The addition of caffeine to the carbohydrate–electrolyte drink resulted in a significant improvement in the performance times as compared to placebo or carbohydrate–electrolyte drink alone, with a maximum effect at an intake of about 3 mg of caffeine per kilogram. There was no apparent change in metabolic fuel used during the cycling exercise, thus ruling out fuel shifts as the mechanism by which caffeine augmented the carbohydrate effect. No caffeine-only treatment was included in this experiment, leaving the question open as to how much of the effect was due to caffeine alone and how much to the interaction of caffeine and carbohydrate.

Sasaki and colleagues (1987) looked at the effect of placebo, sucrose, caffeine (approximately 6 mg/kg of body weight), and a sucrose plus caffeine mixture on time to fatigue in five trained males running at 80 percent VO_{2max}. There was no additive effect of caffeine on time to exhaustion when it was given with sucrose, although the mean distance covered was greater in the two trials where the subjects consumed sucrose compared to placebo. Caffeine alone resulted in a distance intermediate between the two sucrose trials, but it was not significantly different from either. Caffeine alone was associated with an increase in energy derived from fat, whereas sucrose alone was associated with an increased utilization of carbohydrate. Sucrose in combination with caffeine maintained the higher carbohydrate utilization equivalent to sucrose alone. The small number of subjects in this experiment makes it difficult to project these findings to all other populations, including military personnel.

Other Effects on Physical Performance

It has been postulated that caffeine might impinge on physical performance via changes in body temperature and fluid balance. Caffeine apparently has no effect on rectal temperature, plasma volume change, or sweat rate during endurance exercise in warm (25–29°C) environments (Falk et al., 1990; Gordon et al., 1982). No similar studies have been conducted in hotter conditions; however, if an effect is not seen at 25–29°C, it is unlikely that there would be a differential response due to caffeine at temperatures greater than 29°C. Further, a study by Cohen et al. (1996) on performance in a hot and humid environment showed no effect of consuming 5 or 9 mg of caffeine per kilogram on time to exhaustion, body temperature, or blood levels of glucose and lactate during multiple 21-km runs in trained men and women.

High-altitude exposure may augment the positive effects of caffeine on endurance performance. Exercise performance is dramatically reduced by altitude exposure, and maximal effort may be diminished by as much as 25 percent. Submaximal performance may be improved with acclimatization, but maximal effort does not normally recover (IOM, 1996). However, Fulco et al. (1994) showed that ingestion of caffeine (4 mg/kg) could increase the time to exhaustion in eight trained men riding a cycle ergometer at 80 percent of high-altitude VO_{2max} (65 percent of sea-level VO_{2max}) at 4,300 m, but not at sea level. This positive effect was present after 1 hour of altitude exposure (54 percent increase in time to exhaustion with caffeine ingestion 1 hour before exercise) and tended to remain after 2 weeks of acclimatization (24 percent increase). Because Fulco et al. did not find any differences in substrate metabolism between the two conditions, they hypothesized that the mechanism of improvement involved an increase in residual lung capacity (tidal volume) or an improvement in muscle strength. Similarly, Berglund and Hemmingsson (1982) showed that caffeine significantly decreased the race time (by 101 seconds after one lap, 152 seconds after two) of trained cross-country skiers in a 21-km race at 2,900 m. No change in race time occurred in a test at an altitude of 300 m.

A combination of caffeine and ephedrine enhances running performance (Bell and Jacobs, 1999), but also raises metabolic heat production and thus poses a theoretical risk of hyperthermia during exercise–heat stress. However, during 2 hours of brisk treadmill walking in a 40°C hot, dry environment, Bell et al. (1999) observed that this increased metabolic heat production was offset by increased heat dissipation and that the internal body temperature change was no greater than during a control trial. However, recent information on adverse cardiovascular and central nervous system events resulting from the use of ephedra-containing supplements (Haller and Benowitz, 2000) makes the use of a caffeine–ephedra combination less than desirable. Although hyperthermia is more likely when prolonged, strenuous exercise and intense environmental stress are concurrent, the effects of caffeine in this situation have not been examined.

COGNITIVE FUNCTION AND ALERTNESS

Both common experience and the results of scientific investigations support the belief that caffeine enhances performance on a variety of cognitive tasks. However, a review of the experimental literature reveals inconsistencies in the amount of caffeine that is required to produce positive effects on cognitive behavior. These discrepant findings can be explained by differences among experiments in a number of variables including whether or not subjects were tested following a period in which they had abstained from using caffeine, the tasks used to assess cognitive behavior, the age and gender of the subjects, the subjects' history of caffeine use, and whether the subjects were rested or sleep deprived.

There has been some debate whether caffeine enhances cognitive performance or simply restores degraded performance following caffeine withdrawal in rested individuals. James (1994, 1995, 1998) argued that the majority of studies reporting the effects of caffeine in rested subjects studied moderate caffeine consumers (200–300 mg/d) who were required to abstain from caffeine for some period of time prior to cognitive testing (2–24 hr). Abstinence for regular caffeine users could have resulted in symptoms of withdrawal which include headaches, fatigue, and irritability (Griffiths and Mumford, 1995; Griffiths et al., 1990). James (1994, 1995, 1998), hypothesized that comparisons between caffeine and placebo conditions in experiments assessing the effects of caffeine on cognitive behavior could represent a reversal of deteriorated performance. This may be due to caffeine withdrawal in the placebo condition compared to baseline performance in the presence of caffeine.

A clearer picture of caffeine's effects on cognitive function and behavior has begun to emerge, however. Caffeine can enhance performance on some types of cognitive tasks, and some aspects of mood in rested individuals independent of its ability to reverse symptoms of withdrawal and regardless of the background consumption of caffeine. Warburton (1995) demonstrated that caffeine administered in doses of 0, 75, and 150 mg to adult male, nonsmoking, regular caffeine users, without abstinence from caffeine prior to treatment, improved attention, problem solving, and delayed recall and significantly improved mood ratings. Rogers et al. (1995), using caffeine doses of 0, 70, and 250 mg/day in caffeine users (> 200 mg/d) and nonusers (< 15 mg/d), demonstrated that although caffeine withdrawal had a negative effect on mood, it did not appear to affect psychomotor performance. Jarvis (1993) reported results of a large survey study on coffee and tea consumption showing a highly significant dose-response relationship between habitual caffeine intake and psychomotor performance (simple reaction time, choice reaction time, incidental verbal memory, and visuo-spatial reasoning). This report also clearly demonstrates that tolerance to the performance-enhancing effects of caffeine, if it occurs at all, is incomplete with the result that higher daily caffeine consumers tend to perform better than do low consumers (Jarvis, 1993).

Using objective measures of alertness (multiple sleep latency test, visual and auditory vigilance tasks), Zwyghuizen-Doorenbos et al. (1990) demonstrated in rested, moderate (< 250 mg/d) caffeine users that caffeine administered in 250-mg doses twice a day compared to placebo improved daytime alertness and reaction time on auditory vigilance tasks. Kenemans and Lorist (1995), using male and female undergraduate students with an average coffee consumption of 5.9 cups/day, demonstrated that caffeine given in a single dose of 3 mg/kg body weight ($\approx$ 250 mg/day) increased cortical activation, increased sensitivity (rate at which information on stimuli is accumulated), and increased both speed and accuracy of target selection.

Amendola et al. (1998) reported caffeine at doses of 0, 64, 128, and 256 mg/day enhanced accuracy and reduced reaction time on auditory and visual vigilance tasks in a dose-related manner. Moreover, caffeine significantly increased self-reports of vigor and decreased reports of fatigue, depression, and hostility on the Profile of Moods Scale (POMS). Self-assessments of energy levels were also improved by caffeine (Lieberman et al., 1987; Sicard et al., 1996). However, caffeine did not improve long-term memory (list learning), false alarms in an auditory vigilance task, commission of errors in a four-choice reaction time, or motor coordination. In a simulated military situation involving a tedious task that required sustained attention for proficient performance (i.e., sentry duty), caffeine eliminated the vigilance decrement that occurred with increasing time on duty, reduced subjective reports of tiredness, and did not impair rifle firing accuracy (Johnson, 1999). Additionally, in this situation, caffeine increased the number of correct target identifications in both males and females. However, the reason for this differed with gender. With prolonged sentry duty and no caffeine, men were more likely to fire at friendly targets and women were less likely to fire at foes. Caffeine returned both of these deficits to baseline levels (Johnson, 1999).

Thus, caffeine's effects on cognitive function and mood can be detected in rested individuals, both users and nonusers of caffeine, using a variety of standardized tests. Only certain behavioral functions appear to be susceptible to the influence of moderate doses of caffeine (32–256 mg). In particular, it appears that in well-rested individuals, low and moderate doses of caffeine preferentially affect functions related to vigilance (i.e., the ability of the individual to maintain alertness and appropriate responsiveness to the external environment for sustained periods of time), but have limited effects on memory and problem-solving abilities. At high doses caffeine can interfere with performance of tasks requiring fine motor control (Durlach, 1998; Rogers and Dernoncourt, 1998).

The effects of caffeine on cognitive behavior vary according to dose, the subject's experience with caffeine, and gender. In general, low to intermediate doses (100–600 mg) of caffeine are associated with increased alertness, energy, and concentration, while higher doses can lead to anxiety, restlessness, insomnia, and tachycardia (Heishman and Henningfield, 1992, 1994). Individuals who do not consume caffeine on a regular basis appear to be more susceptible to the negative consequences of caffeine than regular consumers. With respect to gender, because of their smaller lean body mass, women may be more affected by a given dose of caffeine than men.

A number of studies have reported on the effect of age on physiological and cognitive responses to caffeine. Arciero et al. (1995) reported that caffeine ingestion (5 mg/kg fat-free mass) increased free fatty acids and tended to increase rate of appearance of fatty acids in younger men (19–26 years old), but not in older men (65–80 years old); while norepinephrine kinetics and fat oxidation were not affected by caffeine in either age group. Arciero et al. (1998) reported on effects of caffeine ingestion (5 mg/kg fat-free mass) on blood pressure, heart rate, norepinephrine kinetics, and behavioral mood in younger and older men. Resting baseline blood pressure was significantly lower for younger men than for older men. Following caffeine ingestion, blood pressure increased significantly above baseline for older men whereas it remained statistically unchanged in younger men. Heart rates in both groups were unaffected by caffeine ingestion. Norepinephrine kinetics (appearance and clearance rates) were not affected by caffeine in either group, although older men had higher norepinephrine concentrations with caffeine. Older men reported declines in feelings of tension and anger following caffeine ingestion, while younger men reported increased feelings of anger.

Rees et al. (1999) examined the interaction of caffeine and age and found that 250 mg of caffeine significantly decreased reaction times in both 20- to 25-year-olds and 50- to 65-year-olds with no effect on word recall. In contrast, Hogervorst et al. (1998) evaluated the effects of 225 mg of caffeine on memory and memory-related processes in three age groups: young (20–34 y), middle-aged (46–54 y), and older (66–74 y). Short-term memory was negatively affected by caffeine in the young group, positively affected in the middle-aged group, and had no effect in the older group. Jarvis (1993), in a large survey study on coffee and tea consumption, found that when results for reaction time tests were categorized by age group (16–34 y, 35–54 y, 55+ y), caffeine intake had a greater performance-enhancing effect for older people (35–54 y, 55+ y) than younger people (16–34 y). The author hypothesized that this greater sensitivity to caffeine in older adults might be due to the fact that older people tend to operate further below their ceiling than do the young. Alternatively, since the survey only measured coffee and tea consumption, the caffeine intake in the young group was more likely to be underestimated due to much heavier cola and soft drink use in this age group (Jarvis, 1993). Amendola et al. (1998), using subjects in two age groups (18–30 y and > 60 y), tested oral caffeine doses of 0, 64, 128, and 256 mg and found a dose-dependent improvement in mood and performance on the modified Wilkinson Auditory Vigilance Task that was not affected by age.

Thus, it would appear that caffeine effects on performance of vigilance types of tasks is independent of age, while caffeine effects on memory-related tasks may be age-dependent.

COMPENSATION OF SLEEP DEPRIVATION IMPAIRMENTS

Effects of Sleep Deprivation on Cognitive Behavior

Military personnel face many situations in which extended wakefulness may be required, including sentry duty, deployment-related activities, air transportation during emergencies, submarine duty, and combat. As part of their duties in these situations, individuals may have to perform complex cognitive tasks. The performance of these tasks is compromised during periods of extended wakefulness. Sleep deprivation leads to a sequence of impairments in cognitive functioning. These impairments include decreases in alertness, decrements in mental performance, reductions in self-reports of vigor, increases in sleepiness and fatigue, and increases in response reaction time (Kautz, 1999; Newhouse et al., 1989; Penetar et al., 1993, 1994; Wyatt, 1999).

A variety of instruments have been used to quantify the effects of sleep deprivation on behavior in controlled-experimental as well as simulated real-world situations. Alertness has been assessed using objective measures such as ambulatory vigilance monitors, visual and auditory vigilance tasks, and subjective measures such as self-reports and questionnaires. Studies using these measures have found that sleep deprivation impairs performance on vigilance tasks and decreases self-reports of alertness (Bonnet and Arand, 1994a,b; Bonnet et al., 1995; Caldwell et al., 1995; Penetar et al., 1993). A number of mental tasks, such as a serial add–subtract test, logical reasoning, mental rotation, perceptual cueing, and memory tests have been used to assess the effects of sleep deprivation on higher cognitive processes. Using these tasks, mental performance deteriorates as a function of sleep deprivation (Bonnet, 1999; Caldwell et al., 1995; Kautz, 1999; Newhouse et al., 1989; Penetar et al., 1993; Smith, 1999; Stickgold, 1999). Of particular significance, sleep deprivation leads to impairments in performance on cognitive tasks that would be encountered in military situations, such as piloting helicopters, fixed-winged aircraft, submarines, or advance warning aircraft; monitoring sonar or radar screens; and sentry duty. Sleep deprivation also affects mood as measured by standard scales such as the POMS and visual analogue scales. More specifically, as subjects become incrasingly sleep-deprived, increases in fatigue, tension, and depression and decreases in vigor are reported (Bonnet, 1999; Caldwell et al., 1995; Kautz, 1999; Newhouse et al., 1989; Penetar et al., 1993; Smith, 1999; Stickgold, 1999). Sleepiness, as assessed by objective measures including latency to sleep, eyelid movements, electroencephalograms, and muscle tone, and subjective measures such as self-report sleepiness scales, increases directly as a function of the amount of sleep deprivation incurred.

Recent advances in the understanding of sleep mechanisms have identified adenosine as a moderator of the sleep-inducing effects of prolonged wakefulness. Studies have shown that extracellular concentrations of adenosine in the cholinergic regions of the basal forebrain increased progressively during prolonged wakefulness and declined slowly during recovery sleep (Porkka-Heiskanen, 1999; Porkka-Heiskanen et al., 1997). Caffeine, as a known antagonist of adenosine, could thus be expected to promote wakefulness by preventing neuronal uptake of the sleep-promoting adenosine.

Two recently identified neuropeptides (orexins A and B, or hypocretins) are produced exclusively by a well-defined group of neurons in the lateral hypothalamus. These unique orexin peptides act directly at axon terminals to stimulate the release of the major inhibitory neurotransmitter, gamma-amino benzoic acid, and the major excitatory neurotransmitter, glutamate. Together, these two neurotransmitters are responsible for almost all fast synaptic activity in the hypothalamus.

Chemelli and colleagues (1999) reported the development of a strain of orexin knockout mice that developed symptoms virtually identical to narcolepsy in humans. To further evaluate the role of orexin in stimulating wakefulness, the antinarcoleptic drug, modafinil (see Chapter 6) or placebo was administered to normal mice. Modafinil strongly activated the orexin neurons in the lateral hypothalamus. No research has yet been reported that examines the effect of caffeine or paraxanthine on orexin neurons.

Restoration of Sleep Deprivation-Induced Cognitive Deficits with Sleep

All of the above-listed decrements in cognitive behavior can best be reversed by reconstituting sleep. There is a dose effect for the restorative effects of sleep duration on cognitive performance (Bonnet, 1999; Bonnet and Arand, 1994b; Bonnet et al., 1995). Any amount of sleep from as little as a 15-minute nap can restore some degree of function, although the longer the sleep episode, the greater the amount of cognitive function restored (Bonnet et al., 1995). Since the drive for sleep is governed by both a homeostatic and a circadian drive, which are interactive (Wyatt, 1999), these factors must be taken into consideration in determining the timing of naps and their effectiveness in reconstituting mental functioning. Naps are effective both prior to (prophylactic naps) and during (restorative naps) a period of sleep deprivation (Bonnet, 1999; Bonnet and Arand, 1994a; Bonnet et al., 1995).

However, in an earlier, well-designed study, Dinges et al. (1987) examined the effects of temporal placement of naps for alertness during a 56-hour period of sleep deprivation. A 2-hour nap was preceded by either 6, 18, 30, 42, or 54 hours of wakefulness. Naps were placed 12 hours apart near the circadian peak or circadian trough. Performance was measured by a visual reaction time test, and mood was assessed using the Stanford Sleepiness Scale (SSS). Results indicated that a nap at any time during the period of sleep deprivation improved reaction time performance but not SSS ratings. The earlier naps (6 and 18 hours into the wakefulness period) yielded better, and longer-lasting reaction time performance improvements which could be detected more than 24 hours after the nap, despite the fact that these naps were comprised of lighter sleep than later naps. Bonnet (1999) also found that quality of sleep differs between prophylactic naps and naps taken during sleep deprivation. Prophylactic naps are associated with longer sleep latencies and less deep sleep than post-deprivation recovery sleep. Dinges et al. (1987) also found circadian placement of naps had no effect on any parameter measured, and concluded that napping prior to a night of sleep loss is more important in meeting subsequent performance demands than is circadian placement of the nap. Napping appears to prevent sleepiness more readily than it permits recovery from sleepiness. In addition, a negative side effect of sleep during a period of sleep deprivation (restorative sleep) is sleep inertia, a short period of mental confusion upon awakening from such naps that can last as long as 30 minutes (Dinges, 1989; Stamph, 1989).

Restoration of Sleep Deprivation-Induced Cognitive Deficits with Caffeine

When sleep is not an option, caffeine can help to alleviate decrements in cognitive functioning resulting from shift work (Walsh et al., 1990, 1995), performance during circadian troughs (Gander et al., 1998; Reyner and Horne, 2000), restricted or disrupted sleep (Belland and Bissell, 1994; Rosenthal et al., 1991), and complete sleep deprivation (Bonnet, 1999; Jarvis, 1993; Johnson, 1999; Kautz, 1999; Lieberman, 1999; Lorist et al., 1994a,b; Smith and Rubin, 1999). The effectiveness of caffeine in reversing sleep deprivation-induced decrements in performance varies among subjects, and its ability to restore mental performance is influenced by a number of factors. These include prior caffeine exposure, dosage schedule, formulation of caffeine, metabolic factors, concurrent drug use, degree of sleep deprivation, and time of day of dose administration

(Kaplan et al., 1997; Kuznicki and Turner, 1986; Linde, 1995; Lorist et al., 1994a,b). From the limited data available, gender does not appear to play a role in the effects of caffeine on mental abilities. However, this variable and other potential factors, such as P450 enzyme polymorphism, age, body weight, stress hormonal and other endocrine responses, concurrent illness, and drug interactions (Kamimori et al., 1999), which might potentially contribute to intra- or intersubject variability to the effects of caffeine, should be assessed further.

In sleep-deprived subjects, judicious use of caffeine can restore alertness, performance on mental tasks, and positive mood states. For example, Smith and Rubin (1999) found that caffeine had a similar profile to amphetamine and phentermine in that it reversed the sleep deprivation-induced increased response time and number of errors on a visual vigilance task, as well as the sleep deprivation-induced decrements in a running memory test. Similarly, Bonnet and Arand (1994b) observed that caffeine increased alertness and performance on a visual vigilance task, mental arithmetic tests, and logical reasoning in sleep-deprived subjects. A number of researchers have shown that caffeine is also effective in delaying sleep onset in sleep-deprived subjects (Bonnet, 1999; Kautz, 1999; Penetar, 1999; Smith, 1999). With respect to mood, caffeine administration in sleep-deprived subjects decreased reports of confusion and fatigue and increased reports of vigor, but had no effect on reports of tension, anger, and depression using the POMS (Kautz, 1999). Using visual analog scales, caffeine intake led to reports of decreased sleepiness and increased alertness, ability to concentrate, confidence, talkativeness, energy levels, anxiety, jitteriness, and nervousness (Kautz, 1999). One study suggested that some of the effects of caffeine were associated with increased measures of hypothalamic–pituitary–adrenal axis activity (plasma cortisol levels). However, further studies utilizing more extensive sampling are needed to confirm this effect.

Research suggests that doses of caffeine between 150 and 600 mg are effective in alleviating sleep deprivation-induced decrements in cognitive performance (Kelley et al., 1996; Penetar et al., 1993). Immediately following administration, doses in the range of 150 mg were just as effective as 300 or 600 mg in improving mental function in sleep-deprived subjects. However, the lower dose (150 mg) did not sustain performance on complex mental operations for as long as the higher doses (300 or 600 mg) (Kautz, 1999). Penetar et al. (1993) administered caffeine at levels of 0, 150, 300, and 600 mg following 49 hours of sleep deprivation and found a dose-related improvement in both subjective and objective measures of alertness and improvements in mood. Kelley et al. (1996) evaluated repeated doses of caffeine during 64 hours of sleep deprivation and measured effects on recovery sleep. Treatments were placebo, 300 mg of caffeine every 6 hours, or 400 mg of caffeine every 24 hours starting the evening of the first day of sleep deprivation. Subjects given the 300 mg every 6 hours developed a steady-state concentration of salivary caffeine by the third dose, while those receiving the 400 mg every 24 hours had salivary caffeine concentrations that peaked and then declined to near placebo level by 18 hours after administration. Caffeine had no effect on recovery sleep with respect to sleep latency, total sleep time, or rapid eye movement sleep. There was actually a nonsignificant increase in slow wave sleep with caffeine compared to placebo.

In comparison to 20 mg of amphetamine however, caffeine's effects are modest. Newhouse et al. (1989) found that 20 mg of amphetamine effectively restored alertness to almost 100 percent of rested values for 2 hours and remained significantly better than placebo for 7 hours after administration. In the Penetar et al. (1993) study caffeine restored alertness to approximately 50 percent of that seen in the rested condition with effects declining after 4.5 hours, although subjective measures of sleepiness following caffeine administration were restored to rested levels for 2 to 12 hours.

Restoration of Sleep Deprivation-Induced Cognitive Deficits with a Combination of Caffeine and Naps

Bonnet and Arand (1994a) compared the effectiveness of a 4-hour prophylactic nap alone to a 4-hour prophylactic nap followed by 200 mg of caffeine during the sleep deprivation period. Results showed that subjects given a combination of a 4-hour prophylactic nap prior to 24 hours of sleep deprivation and 200 mg of caffeine administered at 0130 and 0730 (normal circadian trough) during the sleep deprivation period maintained alertness and performance at levels equal to or better than those demonstrated prior to sleep deprivation, and was significantly better than the 4-hour prophylactic nap alone. In a subsequent study, Bonnet et al. (1995) evaluated differing lengths of prophylactic naps and differing doses of caffeine on performance during sustained operations and found that an 8-hour nap prior to the period of sleep deprivation was most effective in maintaining performance during the first 24 hours without sleep, and that repeated doses of caffeine at 150 or 300 mg every 6 hours were more effective than a single dose of 400 mg. However, neither nap nor caffeine conditions could maintain performance near rested levels beyond 24 hours.

SUMMARY

Caffeine can significantly improve physical performance of an endurance nature. It is unclear at this time whether this is a result of increased production of free fatty acids to spare glycogen or an increase in release of endorphins that permits athletes to exercise longer by altering pain perception. Caffeine may be particularly beneficial in enhancing performance at high altitudes, with or without acclimation. The role of caffeine–carbohydrate combinations in enhancing physical performance still needs to be clarified.

Evidence is presented that caffeine can enhance certain types of cognitive performance, most notably vigilance and reaction times, in rested individuals regardless of whether or not they are regular caffeine users. The response to caffeine in caffeine users has been shown to be over and above any alleviation of withdrawal symptoms.

Sleep is the most effective means of reconstituting the decrements in cognitive functioning brought on by sleep deprivation. Thus, in situations where it is feasible, sleep should be promoted. When naps are not an option, caffeine alone could be used to partially alleviate sleep deprivation-induced impairments in cognitive behavior. Combining naps with judicious caffeine use may be the best remedy for sleep deprivation-induced decrements in cognitive function in military situations where adequate sleep cannot be obtained.

The doses of caffeine most likely to be effective without causing undesirable mood effects are within the range of 100 to 600 mg.

4

Safety of Caffeine Usage

People around the world have been consuming caffeine for more than 1,000 years, but in the United States for at least the last 100 years its use has been surrounded by controversy related to potential negative health and behavioral effects, starting with federal seizure of a shipment of Coca-Cola syrup in October 1909. Among the charges used to support the legality of this seizure was that caffeine was an "added" and "poisonous and deleterious substance".

In 1959 caffeine was listed in the *Code of Federal Regulations* (21 CFR 182.1180—formerly 21 CFR 121.101) as generally recognized as safe (GRAS) when used in cola-type beverages with a tolerance set at 0.02 percent. The tolerance was based on industry practice at that time. The minor food use of caffeine in baked goods, frozen dairy desserts, and so forth is based on independent GRAS determinations.

In 1978 the Select Committee on GRAS Substances of the Federation of American Societies for Experimental Biology completed an evaluation of the safety of caffeine. That committee's conclusions stated that "while no evidence in the available information on caffeine demonstrates a hazard to the public when it is used in cola-type beverages at levels that are now current and in the manner now practiced, uncertainties exist requiring that additional studies should be conducted". The major concern raised in that report was the potential behavioral effect of caffeine, especially in young children.

In 1980 the Food and Drug Administration (FDA) proposed to delete the use of caffeine as an added food ingredient from the GRAS list, to declare that no prior sanction exists for the food use of caffeine, and to list caffeine as a food additive on an interim basis pending the conduct of additional safety studies. The agency identified several safety issues of concern with regard to caffeine, namely potentially fetotoxic and teratogenic properties, potential behavioral effects, and potential carcinogenicity (FDA, 1980b).

In 1987 the FDA published a proposed rule on the use of caffeine in nonalcoholic carbonated beverages. Based on comments submitted to the agency in response to the proposal published in the *Federal Register* of October 1980, the FDA proposed to codify a prior sanction for the use of added caffeine in nonalcoholic carbonated beverages. Thus, the agency was proposing to use a provision of the Food, Drug and Cosmetic Act that exempts from the definition of a food additive any substance used in accordance with an approval granted prior to the Food Additives Amendment of 1958. The FDA concluded that existing data did not demonstrate that a level of 0.02 percent caffeine added to nonalcoholic, carbonated beverages presented any risk to humans. The agency also received several comments regarding the use of caffeine in other foods, but because these comments did not assert that such uses were sanctioned previously, these uses were not addressed in the proposal (FDA, 1987).

In 1992 FDA's Center for Food Safety and Applied Nutrition (CFSAN) carried out a review of scientific articles published from 1986 to 1991 that had bearing on the potential health effects of caffeine. The new information reviewed included animal and clinical studies on developmental, reproductive, behavioral, carcinogenic, cardiovascular, and other effects. Based on this review, CFSAN found that there was no evidence to show a human health hazard arising from the consumption of caffeine through use of cola beverages at 100 mg/person/day or less. The exposures to caffeine from the intake of cola beverages at the ninetieth percentile for children (aged 3 to 5 years) and over a lifetime are estimated by CFSAN to be 57 and 98 mg/person/day, respectively. These daily intakes are within the safe limit set by the prior sanction in 1959. Currently, caffeine is recognized by FDA as a substance that is a food additive with a provisional listing status.

Despite this extensive scrutiny there continues to be controversy surrounding the effects of caffeine on long-term health. The list of diseases in which caffeine has been implicated has changed over the years. Convincing research evidence has removed several diseases from consideration, including various cancers and benign breast disease. Extensive research also has evaluated the impact of caffeine consumption on the incidence of cardiovascular disease, reproduction and pregnancy outcomes, osteoporosis, and fluid homeostasis.

With respect to the actions of caffeine on the central nervous system, it has been shown that ingestion of very high doses of caffeine can produce undesirable effects on mental function such as fatigue, nervousness, and feelings of anger or depression. Additionally, caffeine use has been associated with physical dependence, which may be reflected in performance decrements during withdrawal under some circumstances.

CAFFEINE AND CARDIOVASCULAR DISEASE RISK

For more than 30 years caffeine has been of interest in the etiology of heart disease particularly because it may be associated with alterations in blood lipids and blood pressure, arrhythmias, and other adverse cardiac functions. While earlier studies suggested an effect of caffeine on blood lipids, Sedor et al. (1991) found no influence of coffee on serum lipoproteins in women with normal cholesterol levels. These different results may be accounted for by the finding that the method of preparing coffee could influence the relationship between caffeine and blood lipids. Only one fraction of boiled coffee was found to significantly increase blood cholesterol and low-density cholesterol in a dose-dependent manner (Pirich et al., 1993). In 1,074 adults studied in the United Kingdom, coffee consumption was not found to have a significant effect on total or high-density lipoprotein cholesterol (Lancaster et al., 1994). Similarly, Lewis et al. (1993) found no consistent associations between caffeine-containing beverages and serum lipoproteins in 5,115 healthy black and white, men and women aged 18–30 years. In contrast, in a 17-month follow-up of 2,109 healthy nonsmokers, Wei et al. (1995) found that total serum cholesterol increased by about 2 mg/dL for each subsequent increase in cups of regular coffee per day. Furthermore, a dose–response in serum lipoproteins was found among those who increased consumption, continued the same dose, or decreased consumption of regular coffee. This association was not observed with the consumption of decaffeinated coffee, regular or decaffeinated tea, or caffeine-containing colas. However, in a double-blind, randomized trial of 69 young healthy subjects whose habitual coffee consumption was 5.9 cups (140 mL) of filtered regular coffee per day, abstinence from caffeine resulted in no effect on serum lipids (Bak and Grobbee, 1991). Urgert and Katan (1997), in an extensive review, found effects of coffee brewing techniques on serum concentrations of total and low-density lipoprotein cholesterol. The compounds responsible for this effect are the diterpene lipids cafestol and kahweol, which make up about 1 percent (wt:wt) of coffee beans. These diterpenes are extracted by hot water but are retained by paper filters, thus explaining why filtered coffee has no effect on serum cholesterol, while boiled coffees such as Scandinavian cafetiere and Turkish coffees do.

Several approaches have been utilized to investigate the possible relationship between caffeine intake and blood pressure. Results summarized in recent reviews by Myers (in press) and Green and Suls (1996) suggested that caffeine-naive individuals may experience a small increase in blood pressure after acute dosing with caffeine. During chronic administration of caffeine, tolerance appears to develop, and chronic long-lasting changes in blood pressure are usually not seen in individuals who routinely consume caffeine. Coffee consumption was shown to have no significant effects on blood pressure in the 1,074 adults studied by Lancaster et al. (1994). Similarly, in the Coronary Artery Risk Development in Young Adults study of 5,115 black and white men and women aged 18–30 years, no consistent association was found between consumption of caffeine-containing beverages and blood pressure (Lewis et al., 1993). The 6-year data from the Multiple Risk Factor Intervention Trial showed a significant, independent, inverse relation between caffeine intake and both systolic and diastolic blood pressure (Stamler et al., 1997). In contrast, a recent report of a meta-analysis of 11 controlled trials showed an independent, positive relationship between cups of coffee consumed (median dose = 5 cups/day) and subsequent change in systolic blood pressure (Jee et al., 1999). Another recent review critically examined 30 years of controlled clinical and epidemiological studies on the blood pressure effects of coffee and caffeine (Nurminen et al., 1999). The authors concluded that the acute pressor effects of caffeine are well documented, but that at present there is no clear epidemiological evidence that caffeine consumption is causally related to hypertension. They also concluded, however, that high caffeine intake may be an additional risk factor for hypertension at the individual level due to long-lasting stress or a genetic susceptibility to hypertension.

In general, controlled clinical attempts to demonstrate the effects of caffeine on increasing heart rate or inducing arrhythmias have been unsuccessful (Myers, in press). Chelsky et al. (1990) reported that in patients with clinical ventricular arrhythmias, ingestion of 275 mg of caffeine did not significantly alter the inducibility or severity of arrhythmias. Newby et al. (1996) conducted a randomized, double-blind, 6-week intervention trial using dietary caffeine restriction, caffeinated coffee, and decaffeinated coffee in 13 patients with symptomatic frequent idiopathic ventricular premature beats. Results showed no significant changes in palpitation scores of premature beat frequencies during the intervention weeks and no significant correlation between these variables and serum caffeine concentrations.

A possible association between coffee and risk of coronary heart disease has been examined in case-controlled as well as longitudinal cohort studies. Case-control studies have produced variable results (Myers, in press). However, a meta-analysis of 11 prospective, longitudinal cohort studies showed no increased risk of coronary heart disease associated with consumption of up to 6 cups of coffee per day (Myers and Basinski, 1992). Based on a meta-analysis of 8 case-control studies and 15 cohort studies, Kawachi et al. (1994) reported a pooled case-control odds ratio of 1.63 (95 percent confidence interval [CI], 1.50–1.78) for the effect on coronary heart disease of drinking 5 cups of coffee per day versus none. However, the odds ratio from the 15 cohort studies was not statistically significant. A study of 10,359 men and women in the Scottish Heart Health Study showed a significantly higher prevalence of coronary heart disease in subjects who were nonusers of coffee than in those who drank varying amounts of coffee (Brown et al., 1993). A more recent follow-up of subjects in the Scottish Heart Health Study showed that for many conventional risk factors, coffee had a weak but beneficial gradient with increasing consumption (Woodward and Tunstall-Pedoe, 1999). A 10-year follow-up of North American women participating in a large prospective cohort study showed no evidence for any positive association between coffee consumption and risk of subsequent coronary heart disease (Willett et al., 1996). For women initially drinking 6 cups or more of caffeine-containing coffee per day, the relative risk was 0.95 (95 percent CI, 0.73–1.26) compared to women who did not consume regular coffee.

Despite numerous studies attempting to show a relationship between caffeine and serum lipoproteins, blood pressure, cardiac arrhythmias, and risk of coronary heart disease, results have failed to show a consistent adverse effect of ingestion of moderate amounts of caffeine. Thus, increased risk of cardiovascular problems resulting from the use of caffeine supplements by the military would, in most cases, not appear to be a major concern.

One potential risk should be noted, however. A number of studies have demonstrated that caffeine consumption produces a transient elevation in blood pressure and that this occurs regardless of whether the individual is or is not a habitual user of caffeine (James, 1990; Lane et al., 1990, 1998). Caffeine consumption has also been demonstrated to potentiate the effects of acute exercise and mental stress in increasing blood pressure (Höfer and Bättig, 1993; Lane et al., 1990; Myers et al., 1989). This effect of caffeine is more pronounced in those with high stress reactivity (i.e., high levels of anxiety) and those who are borderline hypertensive or are hypertensive (James, 1990; Lane et al., 1998; Lovallo et al., 1991; Sung et al., 1995). Lovallo et al. (1996) demonstrated that in borderline hypertensive men, the use of caffeine in situations of behavioral stress may elevate blood pressure to a clinically meaningful degree and that these types of blood pressure rises in hypertensives would be large enough to transiently reduce the therapeutic effects of antihypertensive medication. However, earlier work by Greenberg and Shapiro (1987) compared two levels of caffeine in males with or without a family history of hypertension and found systolic blood pressure levels were significantly greater in individuals with a family history of hypertension across all conditions, but not specifically in response to caffeine. Wise et al. (1996) examined the effects of placebo or 6 mg of caffeine per kg lean body mass on calcium metabolism in normotensive and hypertensive individuals. Urinary excretion of calcium over 72 hours following caffeine/placebo dosing was not different with respect to caffeine treatment, or between hypertensive and normotensive subjects. Both Eggertsen et al. (1993) and MacDonald et al. (1991) reported 24-hour ambulatory blood pressures were not different between decaffeinated and caffeinated coffee in treated hypertensives.

Since military scenarios in which the use of caffeine supplements might be desirable would frequently occur when personnel are also under acute mental and/or physical stress, this could be a concern to those personnel with family histories of hypertension.

CAFFEINE EFFECTS ON REPRODUCTION

Caffeine consumption has been suggested as the cause of numerous negative reproductive outcomes, from shortened menstrual cycles to reduced conception, delayed implantation, spontaneous abortions, premature birth, low infant birthweight, and congenital malformations. As with most other aspects of caffeine consumption, there is a paucity of reliable data concerning the metabolic effects of caffeine on reproductive processes. As a general conclusion, no adverse effect on reproduction (e.g., conception, pregnancy, lactation) has been linked consistently to caffeine consumption (Christian and Brent, 2001; Leviton, 1998). Similarly, the effects of small amounts of caffeine on infants and children seem to be modest and typically innocuous (Castellanos and Rapoport, in press). Nevertheless, physicians conventionally recommend that caffeine intake be limited in pregnant women and nursing mothers. This position is also taken by the FDA (Williams, 1999). Such recommendations are in keeping with pharmacological data showing that caffeine is distributed throughout body water, crosses the placenta to enter the fetus, and is secreted in milk.

A number of reviews have examined the association between caffeine consumption and fertility, as well as its effects during pregnancy on risk of premature births, spontaneous abortions, and fetal problems including low birthweight and congenital malformations. In an epidemiological study of 403 healthy premenopausal women, heavy caffeine consumption (more than 300 mg of caffeine per day) was associated with a shortened menstrual cycle, but not with anovulation or short luteal or long follicular phase (Fenster et al., 1999). The conflicting results and methodological inadequacies of some studies surveying the association in humans between caffeine intake and effects on fertility, birthweight, premature births, or congenital malformation (when malformations of all organs is used as the outcome measure) suggest that caffeine has no consistent effect on these outcomes in humans (Leviton, 1993, 1998) despite the findings in animal studies.

Extremely high doses of caffeine in pregnant rats (well outside the range of normal human consumption) are associated with teratogenicity and fetal and maternal loss (Christian and Brent, 2001; Leviton 1993, 1998; Purves and Sullivan, 1993). Similar teratogenic effects have not been confirmed in humans, and the relevance of the route of administration (intraperitoneally) in animal studies is dubious. More recent animal studies, using lower doses of caffeine, have indicated that preconceptual exposure of rats to caffeine reduced fertility due to effects on implantation rather than fertilization rate and was associated with lower birthweight and lower neonatal and prepubertal growth rates (Pollard et al., 1999). Other studies by these same authors have indicated that in rats, caffeine administration during pregnancy is also associated with increased fetal mortality, impaired sexual differentiation, and reduced maturation of neuronal mechanisms controlling respiration and parturition.

Recent reviews of human studies suggest that some of the initial reported associations between caffeine and reduced fertility, teratogenicity, and other fetal and maternal effects in humans may be explained by confounders such as associated cigarette smoking, reporting inaccuracies, and other methodological errors (Christian and Brent, 2001; Leviton, 1998). A prospective study of 210 women consuming moderate and high levels of caffeine showed no association between birthweight of offspring and caffeine consumption (Caan et al., 1998). In contrast, a population-based study of 7,855 live births showed a small but significant increase in the odds ratio for low birthweight and preterm delivery in mothers consuming both caffeinated and decaffeinated coffee, compared to those consuming neither (Eskenazi et al., 1999). Cigarette smoking was controlled in this study; however the authors could not rule out reporting confounders for caffeine consumption. This would seem to imply that some compound in coffee other than caffeine is the potential cause. A recent meta-analysis of studies encompassing 42,988 pregnancies indicated that there was a small but statistically significant increase in risk of spontaneous abortion and low-birthweight babies in pregnant women consuming more than 150 mg of caffeine per day; however, contributing factors such as maternal age, smoking, ethanol use, or other confounders could not be excluded (Fernandes et al., 1998). A recent population-based, case-control study that controlled for confounders showed no effect of caffeine on low birthweight, preterm births, or intrauterine growth retardation (Santos et al., 1998).

Early spontaneous abortions in caffeine-consuming women have been reported in some studies but not others (Dlugosz and Bracken, 1992). Theoretically, early spontaneous abortions could be related to a caffeine-induced depressed production of placental hormones and a vulnerable implantation. On the other hand, pregnancy slows caffeine metabolism and clearance, especially in the last trimester.

One approach to obtaining an objective assessment of caffeine intake and exposure is to use biomarkers such as serum paraxanthine levels. A recent, well-controlled study of 487 women with spontaneous abortions and 2,087 normal controls, in which caffeine exposure was quantitated objectively by serum paraxanthine levels, showed that the mean serum paraxanthine concentration was significantly higher in women who had spontaneous abortions than in controls (752 versus 583 ng/mL). However, the odds ratio for spontaneous abortion was not significantly increased except in subjects with extremely high paraxanthine levels (> 1,845 ng/mL). The authors concluded that moderate consumption of caffeine was not likely to increase the risk of spontaneous abortion (Klebanoff et al., 1999).

Taken together, these studies suggest that the effects of caffeine on pregnancy and fetal health vary according to the route of exposure and dosing schedule in animals, and according to caffeine dose and levels of exposure in both animals and humans. In humans, confounders that may account for many of the observed effects of caffeine in pregnancy include concurrent cigarette smoking, maternal age, ethanol consumption, and inaccuracies in reporting of caffeine consumption.

Early reports of delayed conception in women who chronically consume as little as 100 mg of caffeine per day have been confirmed in some but not all subsequent studies. However, this relationship is often confounded by coexisting cigarette smoking, which does lead to subfecundity. Based on the available evidence, some physicians recommend that caffeine consumption be avoided entirely by women who wish to become pregnant (Jensen et al., 1998; Stanton and Gray, 1995).

In the 1970s caffeine consumption was linked to benign lumps and fibrocystic disease of the breasts. However, extensive subsequent research has failed to establish a causal relationship between caffeine use and either benign or malignant diseases of the breasts. Wolfrom and Welsh (1990) concluded that the scientific literature to that point demonstrated no consistent role of methylxanthines in the etiology of fibrocystic breast disease and no consistent beneficial effect on the disease of reducing or eliminating methylxanthine consumption.

Possible effects on caffeine metabolism that are caused by hormonal changes during the menstrual cycle are unclear and poorly studied. Elimination of caffeine from the diet has been recommended to lessen premenstrual symptomology (Rossignol, 1985), but the evidence for such an effect remains inconclusive.

CAFFEINE EFFECTS ON BONE MINERAL DENSITY

Caffeine consumption has been proposed as a risk factor for osteoporosis. One of the first papers indicating a deleterious effect of caffeine came from the laboratory of Heaney and Recker (1982). Metabolic studies conducted in a large number of middle-aged women showed that caffeine intake contributed to a negative calcium balance. However, the overall loss amounted to less than 5 mg of calcium per cup of coffee. This original observation stimulated several observational studies that examined the possible relationship between caffeine consumption, calcium intake, and various indices of bone health. In the large number of studies that have since been conducted, there appears to be no consistent trend linking caffeine consumption and negative effects on bone mineral density or incidence of fracture. A moderate increase in hip fracture risk was seen in subjects in the Framingham Study who consumed more than 2 cups of coffee or 4 cups of tea per day (Kiel et al., 1990). In a prospective study of a large number of women aged 34–59 years, a positive relation was observed between caffeine intake and risk of hip but not forearm fracture (Hernandez-Avila et al., 1991). In contrast to these findings, more recent studies have failed to show a detrimental effect of caffeine on total bone mineral gain in three groups of teenage women with mean daily intakes of caffeine ranging from 14 to 77 mg (Lloyd et al., 1998), or in college-age women with a mean caffeine intake of 103 mg/day

(Packard and Recker, 1996). No effect of caffeine on hip fracture rates was found in women with coffee intakes of 5 cups or more per day (Tavani et al., 1995). No effect was observed on bone loss in postmenopausal women whose habitual dietary caffeine intake ranged from 0 to 1,400 mg/day (Lloyd et al., 1997) or on bone mineral density in older men (Glynn et al., 1995). Although early experimental studies also indicated a significant effect on acute calcium diuresis (Massey and Hollingbery, 1988; Massey et al., 1989), subsequent work indicated that this acute phase of excretion was compensated by a later decrease in excretion of calcium in the urine (Kynast-Gales and Massey, 1994). Moreover, in contrast to initial studies, later studies found either no significant effect of caffeine on calcium balance (Barger-Lux et al., 1990) or negative balance only in subjects consuming less than about 660 mg of calcium per day, or half of the currently recommended intake of calcium. After a comprehensive evaluation of currently available data, Heaney (in press) concluded that any deleterious effect of caffeine on calcium balance could be offset by only 1 or 2 tablespoons of milk added to coffee and that the real issue of concern is low calcium intake rather than high caffeine intake.

CAFFEINE EFFECTS ON FLUID HOMEOSTASIS

Wemple et al. (1997) found that the consumption of approximately 2,500 mL of a carbohydrate–electrolyte beverage containing caffeine led to a greater mean 3-hour urine output than the carbohydrate–electrolyte drink alone in a resting condition (1,843 mL with caffeine versus 1,411 mL without caffeine). During exercise, however, the difference between treatments was not significant (398 mL in 5.75 hours with caffeine and 490 mL in 5.75 hours without caffeine with 2,200 mL of fluid consumed during exercise). It should be noted that the caffeine dose in this experiment was extremely low (approximately 1 mg/kg) and was not sufficient to produce a positive effect on cycling performance. The fact that urine volume was affected by this dose could be of significance in military situations where significantly higher caffeine doses may be used. Caffeine ingestion is of particular concern in situations where water balance is already in jeopardy, such as in hot or high-altitude environments.

Although moderate- to high-dose caffeine consumption (e.g., 600–900 mg) may increase fluid and electrolyte losses in urine, a normal diet will replace these losses in most military scenarios (Maughan and Leiper, 1994).

Nussberger et al. (1990) administered an oral dose of 250 mg of caffeine to eight healthy subjects and found an increase in diuresis, and increased sodium, potassium, and osmol excretion within 1 hour post-treatment. However, aldosterone and vasopressin concentrations remained unchanged. Neuhauser-Berthold et al. (1997), in a controlled experiment with 12 healthy volunteers, administered enough coffee to provide 642 mg of caffeine in a single day, and monitored fluid homeostasis in comparison with a group with an equal amount of fluid consumption from mineral water only. Subjects given the caffeine had a highly significant increase in 24-hour urine output of 753 ± 532 ml, a corresponding negative fluid balance, and a corresponding decrease in body weight of 0.7 kg. Total body water as measured by bioelectrical impedance decreased by 2.7 percent, and sodium and potassium excretion increased by 66 and 28 percent, respectively. Caffeine use during prolonged operations in hot environments increases the risk of dehydration because such operations involve large sweat losses and/or inadequate fluid and electrolyte intake. The scientific literature indicates that a total body water deficit may (Gonzalez-Alonso et al., 1992; Maughan and Leiper, 1994; Neuhauser-Berthold et al., 1997) or may not (Brouns et al., 1998; Massey and Wise, 1984) occur. The deficit depends on the amount of caffeine consumed, the individual's history of acute and chronic caffeine use, and the total solute load of the beverage plus accompanying meals (Brouns et al., 1998; Wemple et al., 1997).

Finally, a recent study by Kiyohara et al. (1999), in an attempt to determine if serum uric acid concentration could be used as an indicator of increased urination, examined 2,240 Japanese men. They found that men consuming less than 1 cup of coffee per day had a mean serum uric acid concentration of 60 mg/L, while those consuming 5 or more cups of coffee per day had a mean concentration of 56 mg/L.

DETRIMENTAL EFFECTS OF HIGH DOSES OF CAFFEINE

High doses of caffeine can be acutely toxic. Ingestion of caffeine in doses up to 10 g has caused convulsions and vomiting with complete recovery in 6 hours (Dreisbach, 1974). The fatal acute oral dose of caffeine in humans is estimated to be 10–14 g (150–200 mg/kg) (Hodgman, 1998), but numerous factors can alter an individual's sensitivity to caffeine (e.g., smoking, age, prior caffeine status, pregnancy status, concurrent drug use) and thus alter the toxic dose. Doses of 1,000 mg (approximately 15 mg/kg body weight) have generated detrimental side effects, with early symptoms being insomnia, restlessness, and agitation. These symptoms may progress to mild delirium, emesis, and convulsions. Other symptoms can include tachycardia, asystole, and rapid respiration (Kamimori et al., 1999).

One potential risk of high doses of caffeine that needs further substantiation is dose-related decrements in mental functioning (Kaplan et al., 1997; Kuznicki and Turner, 1986; Lieberman, 1999). A number of researchers have found that high doses of caffeine can adversely affect mental performance. Kaplan and colleagues (1997) reported that although a relatively low dose of caffeine (250 mg) produced favorable subjective effects (e.g., elation, pleasantness) and enhanced performance on cognitive tasks in healthy volunteers, higher doses (500 mg) led to less favorable subjective reports (e.g., tension, nervousness, anxiety, restlessness) and less improvement in cognitive performance than placebo. Negative effects may be more pronounced in nonusers than in regular users of caffeine (Kuznicki and Turner, 1986). Excessive intake of caffeine (caffeinism) may be mistaken for anxiety disorder (Benowitz, 1990). Caffeine has been shown to produce anxiety or panic attacks in individuals with agoraphobia or panic disorders, but not in healthy controls (Boulenger et al., 1984; Charney et al., 1985).

Foreman et al. (1989) examined the effects of 0, 125, and 250 mg of caffeine on performance of a numerical version of the Stroop test, which requires sustained vigilance and intense cognitive effort as well as fast responses. Subjects receiving 250 mg of caffeine had significantly slower response times. Streufert et al. (1997) investigated the impact of 400 mg of caffeine in excess of normal consumption by persons who were already moderate to heavy caffeine consumers (400–1,000 mg/day) on performance of complex managerial tasks. Increased caffeine consumption in these individuals had mixed results. Speed of response to incoming information was faster with added caffeine; however, the managers' capacity to utilize opportunity decreased. The authors postulated that increased response speed in association with decreased effectiveness in immediate recall (Warburton, 1995) may have had unfavorable effects on a performance that requires bringing together events and actions that occur across a time dimension.

Effects of Caffeine in the Context of Stress

Among the preexisting variables that may contribute to variations in caffeine sensitivity are baseline levels of stress exposure. Stress may include physical stress (exercise—see Chapter 3), physiological stress (heat stress—see Chapter 3, infection, sleep deprivation), or psychological stress. Stress exposures in the military may be acute or chronic (IOM, 1999). After stress exposure, stress-responsive neurohormonal and neurotransmitter systems are activated, with associated release of the stress hormones corticotropin-releasing hormone, adrenocorticotropic hormone, and cortisol, and the adrenergic neurotransmitters (epinephrine, norepinephrine), which all interact with caffeine. Caffeine also alters the degree of responsiveness of these stress response systems to stressful stimuli (Iancu et al., 1996). For example, caffeine has been shown to increase plasma norepinephrine, to potentiate epinephrine and cortisol stress reactivity to acute psychosocial stress (Lane et al., 1990), and to increase plasma cortisol levels in response to exam stress in medical students (Pincomb et al., 1987). Caffeine also alters measures of autonomic nervous system function, including heart rate, skin conductance, and electrodermal activity (Zahn and Rapoport, 1987). The degree of responsiveness in these studies varied according to previous caffeine consumption (habitual users versus nonusers).

Risks of Caffeine in Combination with Ephedrine and Other Stimulants

The risks of additive effects of caffeine on cardiovascular function in the context of self-dosing with supplement preparations such as ephedrine or yohimbine should be considered when evaluating additional dosing of caffeine. Waluga et al. (1998) found that administration of a combination of caffeine and ephedrine slightly increased systolic blood pressure during exercise, and addition of yohimbine to this combination increased diastolic pressure and heart rate during rest and increased cardiac work load during exercise. Caffeine and ephedrine have also been found to significantly increase heart rate during exercise (Bell and Jacobs, 1999; Bell et al., 1999) and may also transiently increase metabolic heat production (Horton and Geissler, 1996). A recent FDA-requested review related a number of reported adverse cardiovascular and central nervous system events to the use of ephedra-containing supplements (Haller and Benowitz, 2000). White (1999) recently reviewed interactions of caffeine with nicotine, benzodiazepines, and alcohol on behavior.

Physical Dependence and Withdrawal

The use of caffeine by humans is generally not associated with abuse or addiction (Dews et al., in press). Tolerance to some of the physiological effects of caffeine develops when caffeine-containing beverages are consumed regularly. Withdrawal symptoms often occur with the abrupt removal of caffeine from the diet. The frequency of occurrence of withdrawal, as reported in survey studies and clinical trials, varies anywhere from 4 to 100 percent (Goldstein et al., 1965; Griffiths and Woodson, 1988; Griffiths et al., 1986; Naismith et al., 1970; Robertson et al., 1981; Weber et al., 1993). The symptoms of cessation, when they do occur, are not long-lasting.

The signs and symptoms of withdrawal vary widely and can range from mild to severe, following withdrawal from both low and high doses of caffeine (Silverman et al., 1992). These include headaches, drowsiness, irritability, fatigue, low vigor, and flu-like symptoms including myalgia, nausea, and vomiting.

Caffeine acts as a vasoconstrictor of the cerebral arteries, reducing regional blood flow (Cameron et al., 1990; Mathew et al., 1983), including blood flow velocity in the medullar–cerebral artery (Perod et al., 2000). Caffeine withdrawal is associated with electroencephalogram changes (Reeves et al., 1995) and also causes changes in cerebral blood flow leading to vasodilation in high caffeine users that is thought to be associated with a throbbing, vascular-type headache, one of the most commonly observed caffeine withdrawal symptoms (Couturier et al., 1997; Lader, 1999; Mathew and Wilson, 1985).

This withdrawal phenomenon could lead to decrements in performance during military operations and thus should be avoided. Consuming low doses of caffeine (25–50 mg) or slowly tapering the dose of caffeine can prevent withdrawal symptoms (Griffiths and Mumford, 1995).

SUMMARY

Caffeine is approved as a food additive with provisional status by the FDA, thus indicating that the agency concludes there is no evidence of a human health hazard arising from consumption of caffeine added to foods and cola beverages. However, controversy continues with respect to caffeine's role in cardiovascular disease, negative reproductive outcomes, physical dependency and withdrawal, and excessive intake. The preponderance of evidence indicates that the use of caffeine by the military would not place personnel at increased risk of cardiovascular disease. Evidence on the risk of large doses of caffeine for individuals who are hypertensive or borderline hypertensive is inconclusive. For women there may be a small increase in risk of spontaneous abortion in the first trimester of pregnancy. The effects of caffeine on calcium metabolism may be of some concern only for those with very low calcium intakes (less than 50 percent of the current recommended intake). Caffeine can significantly increase 24-hour urine output, and may or may not alter total body water. Therefore, if caffeine supplements are used, emphasis should be placed on adequate fluid consumption, particularly in hot or high-altitude environments.

High doses of caffeine can have a negative effect on mood and cognitive performance, and thus the maximum content of caffeine in the delivery form of choice should not exceed 600 mg. In addition, caffeine potentiates the effects of physical, physiological, and psychological stress. Military personnel who are habitual caffeine consumers should not be denied access to caffeine in order to maximize effects of a caffeine supplement.

5

Doses and Delivery Mechanisms

Numerous studies exist in the scientific literature evaluating the safety and efficacy of caffeine. These studies have used a wide array of caffeine dosages and delivery mechanisms. This chapter briefly reviews that information (see Chapters 3 and 4 for detailed reviews) and provides recommendations on the doses and forms of delivery most appropriate for military purposes.

OPTIMUM CAFFEINE DOSAGE

The effective doses of caffeine vary from individual to individual, depending on a variety of factors including time of day, usual caffeine intake, whether the individual is rested or fatigued, whether they smoke, or whether they use oral contraceptives. Similarly, the response to sleep deprivation also varies between individuals. Caffeine doses experimentally evaluated for their effects on both physical and cognitive performance have ranged from as little as 32 mg of caffeine (Lieberman et al., 1987) to as much as 1,400 mg (Streufert et al., 1997).

Physical Performance

The levels of caffeine that have consistently enhanced endurance performance, as discussed in Chapter 3, range from about 200 to 600 mg. Pasman et al. (1995) evaluated the effects of 0, 5, 9, and 13 mg of caffeine per kg of body weight on endurance performance as measured using a cycle ergometer. These doses were equivalent to approximately 360, 648, and 936 mg of total caffeine.

Caffeine significantly increased time to exhaustion compared to the placebo, and there were no differences between levels of caffeine, thus the 360 mg dose (5 mg/kg) was as effective as the higher doses.

A series of extensive reviews (Dodd et al., 1993; Graham et al., 1994; Spriet, 1995; Tarnopolsky, 1994) of the scientific literature have consistently concluded that caffeine enhances endurance performance in a variety of activities with doses from 2 to 9 mg mg/kg of body weight (approximately 150–650 mg) However, the mechanism by which caffeine improves endurance exercise performance is unclear, and has variously been attributed to increased lipolysis, decreased glycogenolysis, increased secretion of β-endorphins, and decreased plasma potassium concentrations.

Hogervorst and colleagues (1999) examined the effects of 0, 150, 225, and 320 mg of caffeine, administered in a carbohydrate–electrolyte solution, on cognitive performance of endurance-trained athletes before and after strenuous physical exercise. Prior to exercise, 150 mg of caffeine significantly improved delayed memory recall. Exercise alone improved selective attention and both simple and complex motor functions. Immediately following exercise, 225 mg of caffeine significantly improved signal detection efficiency and reaction time.

Cognitive Performance

Numerous studies of the effects of different caffeine dosages on various aspects of cognitive performance have been conducted in both civilian and military settings. For example, Dimpfel et al. (1993) measured the effects of placebo, 200, and 400 mg of caffeine on human electroencephalogram (EEG) patterns at rest and during mental concentration tests. In addition to the finding that the effects of caffeine can be quantified with EEG spectral densities, they also found that subjects achieved the best results on concentration tests when given 200 mg of caffeine. This included both the number of problems solved per unit time and the percentage of correct solutions. Results of treatment with 400 mg of caffeine tended to be below those of the placebo condition. Foreman et al. (1989) compared the effects of placebo, 125, and 250 mg of caffeine on cognitive performance using memory tests and the Stroop test. They found no effect of caffeine on performance in either test, but there was a trend toward fewer words recalled in the short-term memory test with 250 mg of caffeine. However, Lieberman et al. (1987) found improved performance on four-choice reaction time tests and the Wilkinson vigilance test at all levels of caffeine evaluated (0, 32, 64, 128, and 256 mg) with no effect on self-rated feelings of tension or anxiety.

Warburton (1995) examined the effects of 0, 75, and 150 mg of caffeine on attentional, verbal memory, nonverbal working memory, and problem-solving speed and accuracy in 18 men who were regular coffee drinkers (no more than 3 cups/day). Caffeine improved speed and accuracy on attentional tests (visual information processing) in a dose-dependent manner. Similar to the data of

Foreman et al. (1989), there was no effect of caffeine on immediate verbal recall; however there was a dose-related effect of caffeine on delayed verbal recall. Caffeine also significantly improved the accuracy, but not the speed, of problem solving. Rogers et al. (1995) found significant improvement in reaction time with 70 mg of caffeine compared to placebo. Similarly, Lorist and Snel (1997) found that caffeine at 3 mg/kg (210 mg for a 70 kg person) given to habitual users improved reaction time and decreased false alarm rates in selective attention tasks. Streufert et al. (1997) evaluated the effects of 400 mg of caffeine added to regular caffeine consumption in moderate to heavy caffeine users (400–1,000 mg/day) and found faster responses to incoming information.

In sleep-deprived individuals, similar to those engaging in sustained operations, caffeine at levels of approximately 100–600 mg appears to improve performance (e.g., vigilance, mood, higher cognitive functions) with few acute adverse behavioral effects; some of the positive effects may persist for 8–10 hours (Gander et al., 1998; Kuznicki and Turner, 1986; Lieberman, 1999; Mitchell and Redman, 1992; Reyner and Horne, 2000; Rogers et al., 1995; Smith, 1999; Walsh et al., 1990, 1995). Even individuals who do not normally consume caffeine appear to obtain these caffeine-related positive effects.

An earlier report to the military concerning use of caffeine as a performance enhancer (IOM, 1994) indicated that two of the primary issues still needing resolution in providing caffeine to military personnel were the appropriate carrier to provide the supplement and the amount required to achieve the desired benefit in personnel both habituated and nonhabituated to caffeine. The data reviewed in this report indicate that caffeine will improve cognitive performance regardless of habituation status and thus there is no need to have different dose levels. Caffeine doses between 100 and 600 mg that can be self-selected would be adequate for all personnel.

CAFFEINE DELIVERY MECHANISMS

Doses of caffeine could be delivered to military personnel during sustained operations in a variety of ways (e.g., tablet or capsule form, beverage, food, or gum). Each of these forms has advantages and disadvantages. For example, caffeine provided in pill or capsule form may not be as readily absorbed as caffeine in a food or beverage.

Brachtel and Richter (1992), in a letter to the editor of the *Journal of Hepatology*, described a study in which they compared the bioavailability of a base dose of 366 mg of caffeine from intravenous infusion, an oral dose in aqueous solution, and an oral dose as an uncoated tablet. Using the area under the curve of serum concentration over time, the bioavailability of caffeine in tablet form was found to be 80 ± 16 percent, significantly lower than the 100 percent bioavailability for the intravenous and oral aqueous solution methods of delivery. Liguori et al. (1997) compared absorption and subjective effects of 400 mg of caffeine administered in coffee, cola, and capsule form. Using salivary caffeine levels as an indicator, they found that peak increase in saliva levels was similar for coffee and cola, and somewhat lower from capsules. The time to peak saliva levels of caffeine was also similar for coffee and cola (42 and 39 minutes, respectively), but was slower for the capsule (67 minutes).

Because caffeine is commonly consumed in the military (Lieberman, 1999) and most individuals are familiar with its effects, a clearly labeled caffeine product that permits self-dosing to obtain effective dose levels would appear to be appropriate. Such a self-dose might be provided in increments similar to those within the experience of most caffeine users (e.g., 100 mg). For example, a food/energy bar containing a total of 600 mg of added caffeine could be scored in 6 segments of 100 mg each, pills could be provided in doses of 100 mg each, or a pack of chewing gum could contain 100 mg/piece of gum. Caffeine (600 mg) in a beverage would make individual dose control more difficult unless supplied in dehydrated packets of beverage mix containing 100 mg of caffeine per packet to be reconstituted using an individually selected number of packets.

Labeling would permit the few individuals who might experience adverse effects from use of caffeine, or whose religious beliefs precluded its use, to avoid it. The advantage of food or beverage delivery of caffeine is that it permits simultaneous provision of nutrients (e.g., water), consumption of which may otherwise be inadequate under the stress of sustained operations. Food or beverage delivery also provides the ability to include substances that may potentiate the effects of caffeine (e.g., sugar). Since caffeine is a diuretic, beverages may have a particular advantage in situations in which dehydration is likely. However, adherence to appropriate behavioral directives (e.g., adequate consumption of food and beverages) can reduce this risk.

Sustained operations vary in their operational constraints. In aviation missions, for example, low weight and compactness of the caffeine delivery mechanism (e.g., pills, gum) may have advantages over beverages and food bars, yet beverages and bars have the advantage of providing additional fluid and nutrients. Beverages have some advantages in certain situations. For example, dehydration at altitude is often a problem, and the beverage delivery system lessens this hazard; however, under these conditions thirst may not be sufficient to ensure that an effective caffeine dose is consumed (IOM, 1996). In addition, use of a caffeinated beverage, while light in weight if dehydrated, would require time and a water source for mixing, thus making it a less viable alternative than gum or a food bar. Food/energy bars have the advantage over beverages in their ability to deliver a wider variety of other needed nutrients at equal weight; this is an important consideration in many missions. Pills and gums are both very light in weight and small in size, so they can easily be carried in pockets; gum has the advantage of stimulating salivation and enhancing the speed of absorption. It may be necessary to consider at least two caffeine delivery systems: food bars and gum. Both can be manufactured to provide multiple doses in a single package so that the individual can easily customize his or her optimal effective dose. There is some advantage in having caffeine increments constant at 100 mg (e.g., the score on the bar or the contents of one stick of gum should deliver the same dose) regardless of the delivery mechanism, so that the various forms are more or less interchangeable for self-dosing purposes.

Often sustained operations missions must be altered with little advance notice. In the committee's judgment, it is important that the caffeine delivered be absorbed and metabolized rapidly so that the beneficial effects on performance are present within an hour after administration. Moreover, the dose should not be released over a long time interval because beneficial effects may be delayed and changes in mission cannot easily be accommodated. Information presented in the previous chapters suggests that repeated caffeine dosing during sleep deprivation does not interfere with recovery sleep, suggesting little benefit other than convenience to sustained-release preparations over large single doses (Prusaczyk, 1999). More frequent dosing with rapidly absorbed and metabolized forms of caffeine therefore appears to offer advantages over sustained-release preparations.

SUMMARY

Caffeine has been consistently found to enhance physical endurance performance when administered in amounts ranging from 150 to 650 mg. Similar amounts have also been found to enhance cognitive performance. Caffeine may be administered in a variety of ways, including as a pill or capsule, in a food bar, in a beverage, and in chewing gum. Delivery of caffeine in a food bar or as chewing gum appears to be most advantageous.

6

Special Considerations

In light of wide-ranging individual differences in caffeine sensitivity, dosing for optimal efficacy and minimal side effects should take into account qualitative conditions based on trait and state variations in individual sensitivity to caffeine. Trait variations are those based on the individual's genetic makeup and include such factors as stress reactivity, rate of metabolism of caffeine to paraxanthine, and kidney clearance rates. State variability factors include preexisting caffeine intake from other sources (beverages, foods, supplements), other stimulant drug intake (ephedrine, over-the-counter, or prescription drugs), other drug or hormone use (e.g., oral contraceptives), smoking, stress (heat stress, exercise, other stress), sleep deprivation status, and relevant health conditions (e.g., hypertension, anxiety disorder).

Ideally, a composite quantitative dosing scale (composite caffeine intake index) could be developed using parametric analysis to take into account differences in state and trait variations in individual sensitivity to caffeine. Such a scale could be applied to determine more quantitatively the amount of caffeine that should be administered to individuals in specific contexts for improvements in cognitive function with minimal side effects based on individual differences in preexisting trait sensitivity as well as state variability factors.

If the military adopts the use of caffeine to preserve cognitive performance and vigilance in special and sustained operations, consideration should be given to soldiers' information needs as well as to potential safety issues and ethical concerns. An order to use caffeine may be appropriate to ensure the safety of personnel and the success of a military operation. The committee endorses the concept that the command structure at the lowest level should have the authority to require the consumption of caffeine if, in their judgment, the welfare of the war fighters or the success of a mission would otherwise be at risk. Nevertheless, the dosage of caffeine should include some element of individual choice. That is, the individual should be permitted to control the intake of caffeine much like the civilian population does when consuming coffee or caffeine-containing soft drinks, on the basis of perceived need to sustain performance.

EDUCATION AND TRAINING ISSUES

An education or information component should be a crucial part of any program to provide military personnel with caffeine in order to facilitate an informed decision process. This information component should include potential benefits, methods of implementation including the timing and the dose that may be effective, potential dangers of misuse, physiological symptoms of excessive intake, and the potential dependence (and subsequent withdrawal symptoms) associated with continued moderate to high levels of use. This information component should also include opportunities for consumption of products that contain added caffeine in a controlled situation so that each individual will be aware of how a product impacts his or her own performance and mood prior to use in an operational situation.

Training of command personnel is also essential to assist them in making decisions about when the products are appropriate to use, directions for their use, and any potential adverse effects resulting from misuse.

LABELING

Any nontraditional product that is used as a vehicle for providing caffeine to military personnel (particularly if it could possibly reach civilian hands) should be prominently labeled, including on the principal display panel, that the product contains added caffeine and is intended for use only during sustained or special operations. The label should also contain the amount of caffeine per recommended serving (e.g., stick of gum) and the total amount per package or container. Appropriate doses should be clearly labeled and the product (e.g., chewing gum, food/energy bar, or tablet) should be scored or metered to facilitate obtaining a certain dose (e.g., 100 mg).

The Food and Drug Administration (FDA) has determined that there is no evidence to show a human health hazard arising from the use of caffeine and has approved its use as a food additive with a provisional listing status. Thus the committee believes that a warning statement is not necessary and could lead to unnecessary concern on the part of military personnel instructed to use the product. However, prominent information statements on the misuse of the product are needed. For example, it is recommended that the label display instructions for use that provide the maximum single dose and the frequency of dosing.

ETHICAL CONSIDERATIONS

The committee has deliberated the potential ethical issues associated with the use of caffeine or other stimulants in military operations. In the committee's judgment, it is unethical to coerce any individual to consume caffeine, if for religious or health reasons that individual does not wish to consume stimulants. The committee is aware that it is the military custom for the individual and his or her superior to discuss concerns of this nature and secure consultation of the unit's surgeon if a waiver is necessary.

There are also ethical concerns when caffeine, which is a legal and acceptable substance in American society, is denied in the course of a military operation simply because of a logistical decision. In such situations heavy users are likely to undergo withdrawal symptoms and may put themselves and other war fighters at increased risk due to fatigue, sleepiness, loss of attentiveness, and other withdrawal symptoms.

Although clinical studies do not provide evidence of acute side effects from caffeine consumption in the range under consideration, there seems to be an abundance of anecdotal information that some individuals have significant discomfort when consuming levels of caffeine equivalent to that found in 1 cup of coffee. It is recommended that research be done with volunteers who have been so identified to determine if there is a small segment of the population that may have an increased sensitivity to caffeine.

ALTERNATIVES TO CAFFEINE FOR MAINTENANCE OF COGNITIVE PERFORMANCE

There are a number of possible alternatives to caffeine for maintaining cognitive performance during sustained operations. These include naps and the use of various prescription drugs, which are discussed below.

Naps

Decrements in cognitive behavior due to sleep deprivation can best be reversed by providing sleep. There is a dose effect for the restorative effects of sleep on cognitive performance (Bonnet, 1999; Bonnet and Arand, 1994a; Bonnet et al., 1995). Any amount of sleep from as little as a 15-minute nap can restore some degree of function, although the longer the sleep episode, the greater the amount of cognitive function restored (Bonnet et al., 1995). Since the drive for sleep is governed both by a homeostatic drive and a circadian drive, which are interactive (Wyatt, 1999), these factors must be taken into consideration in determining the timing of naps and their effectiveness in reconstituting mental functioning. Naps are effective both prior to (prophylactic naps) and during (restorative naps) a period of sleep deprivation (Bonnet, 1999; Bonnet and Arand, 1994b; Bonnet et al., 1995). However, the quality of sleep differs between prophylactic naps and naps taken during sleep deprivation. Despite the fact that prophylactic naps are associated with longer sleep latencies and less deep sleep than post-deprivation recovery sleep (Bonnet, 1999), studies by Dinges et al. (1987) demonstrated that prophylactic naps were more beneficial than restorative naps. They concluded that napping prior to a period of extended wakefulness was more important than circadian placement of the nap. A negative side effect of naps during a period of sleep deprivation (restorative naps) is sleep inertia, a short period of mental confusion upon awakening which can last as long as 30 minutes.

A combination of caffeine and naps is the most effective nonprescription drug alternative to caffeine administration alone when a normal sleep regimen is not possible. In a series of studies (Bonnet 1993; Bonnet et al., 1995; Horne and Reyner, 1996) the combination of a short nap and caffeine significantly decreased driving impairment, subjective sleepiness, and drowsiness as measured by electroencephalogram (EEG) activity. The combination of a nap and caffeine also increased alertness during long periods of sleep deprivation compared to either caffeine or naps alone. Thus wherever possible commanders should incorporate strategies that can provide short naps with the use of caffeine for maintaining vigilance, alertness, and other physiological and cognitive functions that are needed for sustained operations (SUSOPS). Placement of the nap as early as possible in the sleep deprivation period, followed by caffeine administration during circadian troughs, would be most effective (Bonnet et al., 1995).

A number of potential alternatives to caffeine (other than sleep) for maintenance of cognitive performance were examined. The use of stimulants, other than caffeine, most frequently referred to in the scientific literature were the drugs pemoline, modafinil, and dextroamphetamine. Although methylphenidate, a drug very similar to amphetamine, is mentioned below, no studies were found in which it was used to enhance or maintain cognitive performance in normal, healthy individuals.

Pemoline

Pemoline is a central nervous system (CNS) stimulant structurally dissimilar from the amphetamines and methylphenidate. It is an oxizolidine compound with poor aqueous and lipid solubility. It is absorbed slowly from the gastrointestinal tract and, in adults, reaches peak plasma concentrations within 2 to 4 hours of administration. The half-life is about 11 to 12 hours, and more than 90 percent of an oral dose is excreted in the urine, with 40 to 50 percent excreted as unchanged drug (Anonymous, 1992b; Sallee et al., 1992; Vermeulen et al.,

1979). Pemoline has a pharmacological activity similar to other CNS stimulants but with minimal sympathomimetic effects. Although the exact mechanism of action is not known, pemoline may act through dopaminergic mechanisms (Molina and Orsinger, 1990; Nicholson and Pascoe, 1989).

Until around 1990 the primary indication for this drug was as a treatment for attention deficit disorder in children and adolescents. However, due to the considerable individual variation in onset and duration of action, its use was secondary to that of methylphenidate and d-amphetamine. Subsequently, it has also been evaluated for the treatment of narcolepsy and excessive daytime sleepiness (EDS).

Since 1990 pemoline has been investigated, primarily by the British Royal Air Force, as a means of maintaining cognitive function during intensive and sustained military operations. Effects of pemoline on cognitive performance during 64 hours of sleep deprivation (Babkoff et al., 1992; Gomez et al., 1993) varied depending on the administration protocol. With single-dose administration, pemoline improved performance on Matrix Pattern Recognition and a tapping test, but had no effect on the speed of reaction. However, on a maintenance protocol (pemoline administered every 12 hours during 64 hours of sleep deprivation), there was less effect on accuracy but a significant improvement in speed of response. Naitoh et al. (1992) compared the effects of prophylactic naps, no naps, pemoline (37.5 mg every 12 hours for a total dose of 200 mg), and placebo during a continuous 64-hour work period. Changes in performance were measured with a four-choice serial reaction time test. Significant benefits in counteracting fatigue and sleep loss were found both for naps and for pemoline, with pemoline showing only a minimal loss in reaction time compared to the no-nap and placebo groups.

Nicholson and Turner (1998) evaluated the effects of pemoline at doses of 10, 20, 30, and 40 mg on subjective alertness of volunteers during a 12-hour overnight work period, using a battery of cognitive function tests. A 6-hour prework sleep period and a 4-hour recovery sleep period were monitored. Pemoline significantly improved subject alertness and performance on all tasks except mental arithmetic and first basic reaction time compared with placebo. The first effects of pemoline were observed 4.5 hours after ingestion for the highest dose on digit symbol substitution and sustained attention reaction time. Positive effects of the lower doses were not seen until 6 hours postingestion, and maximal effects of the drug occurred 9 hours post-ingestion. Both the 30- and 40-mg doses impaired recovery sleep.

Pemoline appears to have limited abuse or dependence potential. In animal studies, pemoline was not self-administered, either in naive or in cocaine-dependent animals (Langer et al., 1986). However, an earlier study by Nicholson et al. (1980) found that 60 or 100 mg of pemoline significantly reduced sleep duration and percentage of rapid eye movement (REM) sleep, and increased the delay to the first REM period. Both doses shortened and fragmented sleep.

Adverse effects that have been most frequently reported from the use of pemoline include hepatic dysfunction and dyskinetic movements of tongue, lips, face, and extremities.

The onset of beneficial cognitive effects from pemoline is quite slow, ranging from 6 to 9 hours postingestion for 10-, 20-, and 30-mg doses. Higher doses have a more rapid onset but also interfere with recovery sleep. Plasma clearance rates are also relatively slow, with a half-life of 11–12 hours. In addition, it is recommended that liver function tests be conducted prior to the use of pemoline because of potential side effects of the drug. Results published to date on aspects of cognitive performance improved by pemoline are confusing.

Modafinil

Modafinil is a benzhydrylsulfinylacetamide derivative first synthesized and produced in France in 1986 as a treatment for narcolepsy that would achieve alertness effects equivalent to those of amphetamine but without impairment of sleep. In the United States modafinil was designated as an orphan drug (for the treatment of EDS in patients with narcolepsy) in 1993. It was approved by FDA for this purpose in 1998, and is classified as a Schedule IV controlled substance (FDA, 1999).

Absorption of modafinil occurs at a rate similar to that of pemoline, with peak plasma concentrations occurring 2–4 hours after oral administration and increasing linearly with doses from 200 to 600 mg. The extent of modafinil absorption was not significantly affected by the presence of food, but the rate of absorption was slightly reduced in fed versus fasted subjects (Moachon et al., 1996). Modafinil has low aqueous solubility and approximately 60 percent is bound to serum proteins, primarily albumin. It is metabolized extensively by the liver to inactive metabolites, modafinil acid (primary form), and modafinil sulfone. The plasma half-life of modafinil after 7 days of dosing was 9–14 hours. Modafinil is excreted in the urine primarily as modafinil acid; only about 10 percent of the dose is excreted unchanged (Moachon et al., 1996).

The mechanism of action of modafinil has not been clearly established, but evidence suggests that it may indirectly increase wakefulness, at least in part, by decreasing gamma-aminobutyric acid-mediated neurotransmission (McClellan and Spencer, 1998), or increasing the secretion of the neuropeptide orexin (Chemelli et al., 1999). Modafinil induces wakefulness and increases locomotor activity in a variety of animal species without causing stereotyped behaviors (Hermant et al., 1991; Lin et al., 1992; Nicolaidis and De Saint Hilaire, 1993). Evidence suggests that the site of action of modafinil differs from that of amphetamines and methylphenidate (Lin et al., 1996), and studies in rats have indicated a potential mechanism of action for modafinil through the stimulation of excitatory amino acids in the cerebral cortex (Piérard et al., 1995). Edgar and Seidel (1997) compared the effects of equivalent doses of modafinil and amphetamine on wakefulness and motor activity in rats and found that modafinil was equal to amphetamine in potently promoting wake time, but did not increase locomotor activity or produce rebound hypersomnolence. The authors concluded that the specificity of modafinil's wake-promoting effects further differentiated it from classical psychomotor stimulants such as amphetamine and methylphenidate.

In a study with cocaine stimulus-trained monkeys and rats, Gold and Balster (1996) evaluated the abuse potential of modafinil, using amphetamine and ephedrine as positive controls. In both rats and monkeys, modafinil did exhibit reinforcing and discriminative stimulus effects, but only at the highest doses tested (0.3 mg/kg). Modafinil was over 200 times less potent than amphetamine and was also less potent than ephedrine.

Broughton and coworkers (1997) compared the effectiveness of placebo to 200 or 400 mg of modafinil in 75 patients meeting international diagnostic criteria for narcolepsy. Compared to placebo, modafinil significantly increased mean sleep latency, with no significant difference between the two doses. Modafinil also reduced the number of daytime sleep episodes and periods of severe sleepiness without interfering with nocturnal sleep initiation, maintenance, or architecture. There were also no changes in blood pressure or heart rate in either normotensive or hypertensive patients. The 400-mg dose of modafinil was associated with increased reports of nausea and nervousness compared to placebo or the 200-mg dose.

A number of studies have examined the effects of modafinil on cognitive performance and sleep recovery in sleep-deprived, but otherwise healthy, volunteers. Modafinil (300 mg) was as effective as 20 mg of dextroamphetamine in maintaining both subjective estimates of mood and fatigue and objective measures of reaction time, logical reasoning, and short-term memory when administered three times during 64 hours of sleep deprivation (Pigeau et al., 1995). Effects on recovery sleep were also monitored in this study, and results indicated that the effects of amphetamine on recovery sleep were similar to those reported previously, with increased sleep latency, decreased total sleep time, decreased REM sleep, and reduced sleep efficiency. Results from the modafinil group exhibited decreased time in bed and sleep period time, with fewer sleep disturbances during the first night of recovery sleep compared to the amphetamine group. There was no effect of modafinil on REM sleep during the first night of recovery sleep, and the second night of recovery sleep did not differ from placebo. Thus, modafinil allowed sleep to occur, displayed sleep patterns close to placebo, and decreased the need for a long recovery sleep to compensate for total sleep deprivation (Buguet et al., 1995). Stivalet et al. (1998) compared the effects of 300 mg of modafinil every 24 hours to placebo in healthy individuals during 60 hours of sleep deprivation. This experiment used the visual search paradigm for assessing speed and accuracy in target detection. Rapid search rates remained unchanged for placebo and modafinil; however, slow search rates increased linearly in the placebo condition with increasing time without sleep, but remained the same as rested controls with modafinil. The number of errors also increased with placebo but remained the same for modafinil. Batejat and Lagarde (1999) examined the effects of 200 mg of modafinil in conjunction with naps on performance during two 27-hour periods of sleep deprivation. The effects of modafinil on cognitive performance during sleep deprivation suggested the compound may act at two levels. First, modafinil maintains an efficient level of CNS general activation close to awakening, and second, it seems also to have a more specific action on neurophysiological mechanisms underlying short-term memory. As in previous studies, modafinil did not prevent sleep if sleep opportunities were available.

Caldwell and coworkers (1999) recently reported on the use of modafinil in a helicopter simulator study with pilots exposed to two 40-hour periods of sleep deprivation. Three 200-mg doses of modafinil or placebo were administered during the 40-hour period. Modafinil significantly attenuated the effects of sleep deprivation on four of six flight maneuvers: straight and levels, straight descent, left standard-rate turns, and left descending turns, maintaining them at baseline levels. Modafinil also reduced the amount of slow-wave EEG activity (indicative of reduced CNS activation), lessened self-reported problems with mood and alertness, and curtailed the performance decrements that were found with placebo. According to these researchers, the most noticeable benefit of the drug was seen when the combined impact of sleep loss and circadian trough was most severe. As in other studies, no disruptions in recovery sleep architecture were observed.

Compared with other well-known stimulatory substances such as caffeine and amphetamine, modafinil appears to have the advantage of combining wakening and stimulating properties, with an appreciable absence of unwanted side effects.

Modafinil does appear to have some abuse potential at high doses, but it was 200 times less potent than amphetamines in this regard. Modafinil has been used as long as 3 years in the treatment of narcolepsy without signs of drug dependence. No toxic effects of high levels of modafinil have been observed in animals.

A dose of 200 mg appears to be quite effective as a single dose for short periods (24 hours) of no sleep or repeated at 12-hour intervals during long periods of sleep deprivation. Maximum effectiveness occurs about 4 hours postingestion and is most beneficial when modafinil is administered during circadian troughs.

Amphetamine

Amphetamines are sympathomimetic amines with CNS stimulant activity. CNS effects are mediated by release of norepinephrine from central noradrenergic neurons. At higher doses, dopamine may be released in the mesolimbic system. Peripheral alpha- and beta-adrenergic activity includes elevation of systolic and diastolic blood pressures and weak bronchodilator and respiratory stimulant activity.

Following oral administration, amphetamines are completely absorbed within 3 hours and widely distributed throughout the body with high concentrations in the brain. Peak plasma levels may occur within 2–3 hours, and maximum effects are reported in the second hour (Angrist et al., 1987).

Amphetamine is metabolized in the liver by aromatic hydroxylation, N-dealkylation, and deamination. Urinary excretion of the unchanged drug is pH-dependent. Urinary acidification to pH below 5.6 yields a plasma half-life of 7–8 hours; alkalinization increases half-life (18–34 hours). For every one unit increase in urinary pH, there is an average 7-hour increase in plasma half-life (Anonymous, 1992a). Although the elimination half-life of amphetamines normally exceeds 10 hours, its behavioral and subjective effects show a clear decline after 4 hours (Angrist et al., 1987).

Studies of the effects of amphetamines on human performance began over 60 years ago. Reviews of the effects of amphetamines on daytime alertness of well-rested subjects show conflicting results. Overall, well-rested individuals appear to benefit little from amphetamines (Spiegel, 1979).

In situations of reduced alertness (e.g., sleep deprivation, night work, sustained-attention tasks), amphetamines have proven to be potent in reversing or preventing performance decrements (Akerstedt and Ficca, 1997). Newhouse et al. (1989) evaluated the effects of placebo, 5, 10, or 20 mg of d-amphetamine during 60 hours of sleep deprivation. The drug was administered 48 hours into the deprivation period, after which sleep latency, behavioral parameters, and cognitive performance were measured. The 20-mg dose returned sleep latency to baseline for 7 hours postadministration. It also improved accuracy on attentional arithmetic tests and improved performance on verbal reasoning tasks. The lower doses were less effective.

In extensive helicopter simulator and in-flight testing, 10 mg of d-amphetamine was observed by investigators (Caldwell and Caldwell, 1997; Caldwell et al., 1995, 2000) to "improve subjective feelings of fatigue, confusion, and depression while increasing feelings of vigor" compared to placebo during 40 hours of sleep deprivation. Amphetamine improved performance of flight maneuvers both in a flight simulator and in actual test flights. Performance was most noticeably improved in the early morning hours following 24 hours of sleep deprivation. Both EEG data and mood ratings showed that alertness was significantly maintained with amphetamine. In a comprehensive follow-up study, Caldwell et al. (2000) administered 10 mg d-amphetamine or placebo three times on each of two sleep-deprivation days (a total of 64 hours of sleep deprivation). Amphetamine sustained flight performance, physiological arousal, and mood throughout the 64-hour period. There were no clinically significant side effects attributable to amphetamine. Some of the aviators complained of palpitations and "jitteriness" with amphetamine, but this did not detract from their flight performance.

In another study of 64 hours of sleep deprivation with 40 subjects in a continuous work environment, 20 mg of *d*-amphetamine, administered on three occasions during the period, significantly improved objective measures of reaction time, logical reasoning, and short-term memory (Pigeau et al., 1995).

All of these studies have demonstrated serious impacts of amphetamine on recovery sleep. At least two uninterrupted 8-hour nights of recovery sleep were needed (Buguet et al., 1995; Caldwell et al., 2000). Amphetamine reduces the amount of REM sleep and reduces sleep efficiency.

Because of the powerful effects of low doses of amphetamine against sleep loss, the military has had considerable interest in the use of amphetamines in sustained operations.

This interest is not new, however. Stimulants were used by both British and German aviators during World War II. Senechal (1988) reported on the use of amphetamine by British Royal Air Force pilots in connection with the Libyan air strike. Emonson and Vanderbeek (1995) reported on the incidence and effectiveness of amphetamine use by U.S. Air Force pilots during operations Desert Shield and Desert Storm. Both the U.S. Air Force (2001) and the U.S. Navy (2000) currently have official memoranda and protocols in place that provide detailed guidance on the use of amphetamines by aviators during continuous operations.

Amphetamine is a controlled substance and thus requires an individual medical evaluation to determine risk factors and health status before a prescription can be issued. Nevertheless, it is possible with appropriate supervision and control that amphetamine could show promise of providing benefits to individuals with unique skills whose performance is critical to the safety of military personnel and complex military hardware.

Amphetamines are very effective in maintaining alertness, cognitive performance, and mood during extended periods of sleep deprivation. These effects can be achieved at low doses (5–10 mg) where adverse side effects are minimal or nonexistent. The military has considerable experience in the use of this stimulant in combat operations, and both the Navy and the Air Force have protocols for use already in place. To date, this use has been restricted to aviators during sustained flight operations.

Amphetamine has a pronounced detrimental effect on recovery sleep that can last two or more nights. In contrast to caffeine in food, beverages, chewing gum, and pill or tablet form, most military personnel have little experience with amphetamine pill self-dosing and the hazards and adverse effects of self-dosing might therefore be expected to be greater. For all the armed services it would be preferable if maintenance of cognitive performance can be achieved without such substances. The potential for abuse of amphetamines is considerable, and appropriately monitoring its dispensing and use may add unnecessary burdens to personnel in the intense and demanding tasks that are directly involved in guaranteeing the success of SUSOPS. Although amphetamine (10 or 20 mg) was more effective in reversing the negative effects of sleep deprivation on alertness than caffeine at doses of 300 mg, it had deleterious effects on recovery sleep, which may also be important in the ultimate success of demanding and constantly changing SUSOPS (Bray et al., 1999). Amphetamine should not be considered a substitute for sleep, and more nights of recovery sleep are needed after its administration (Caldwell, 1999). Therefore, considerable caution is warranted, and use of this stimulant should be restricted to only those extreme circumstances when such measures are considered essential to the success of highly sensitive operations.

The use of modafinil in place of amphetamines under these special circumstances should be explored thoroughly. Research to date indicates that the potential for abuse of modafinil is considerably less than for amphetamines (about 200 times less), and modafinil does not affect initiation of recovery sleep. The committee recommends that modafinil receive more evaluation in simulated military operations before operational testing of the drug.

Prescription drugs in the United States can be prescribed for off-label uses by physicians. In the case of modafinil, which is approved as a wakefulness-promoting drug, its use in healthy individuals as opposed to narcoleptics would be an off-label use. However, there is ample precedence for off-label use of drugs by military medical personnel, as in the limited prescription of dextroamphetamine to pilots on long-range missions and the use of pyridostigmine bromide as a pretreatment to protect troops from the harmful effects of nerve agents during the Gulf War.

SUMMARY

Any program designed to provide caffeine to military personnel should allow individual control of dosage and include an education and training component. Personnel should have the opportunity to experience the dose to be used in a nonoperational situation. Commanders should be advised of when caffeine use is appropriate as well as signs of adverse effects due to excessive dosing. Caffeine-supplemented products should be clearly labeled as such, along with instructions for use.

Ethical considerations would include the question of forcing caffeine use when an individual has strong religious or health reasons for not doing so. Conversely, denying access to caffeine for habituated users either for logistical reasons or in expectation of a subsequent need for a caffeine supplement could risk decrements in performance due to caffeine withdrawal.

Alternatives to caffeine for maintaining cognitive performance include use of naps or prescription drugs. The prescription drugs that have been evaluated for use in healthy adults undergoing sleep deprivation are pemoline, amphetamine, and modafinil. Of these three compounds, modafinil and amphetamine have been shown to be superior to pemoline. Modafinil is as effective as amphetamine, but does not interfere with recovery sleep and has significantly less potential for abuse.

7

Response to Military Questions, Conclusions, and Recommendations

This chapter presents the committee's responses to the specific questions posed by the military by briefly reviewing the pertinent information provided in the earlier chapters. It then presents the committee's conclusions and recommendations.

1. Efficacy: Does the Committee on Military Nutrition Research stand by its earlier recommendation that there are sufficient data to recommend a caffeine product to enhance performance? What are the specific indications for use and contraindications for use?

Caffeine has been shown to induce a variety of positive effects that have contributed to its extensive use worldwide. Caffeine use has been associated with enhanced physical performance and increased alertness, and as a countermeasure to the effects of sleep deprivation. Extensive research has been done on each of these caffeine effects.

Caffeine use is associated with a reproducible increase in endurance time in physical activities of moderate intensity and long duration. Caffeine enhances endurance performance in a variety of activities (i.e., running, cross-country skiing, cycling), with doses in the range of 2 to 9 mg/kg (approximately 150–650 mg in a 70–72 kg individual), in both naive and habituated, trained and untrained, test subjects. High-altitude exposure may augment the positive effects of caffeine on endurance performance. Exercise performance is dramatically reduced by altitude exposure, and maximal effort may be diminished by as much as 25 percent. Ingestion of caffeine (4 mg/kg) increased the time to exhaustion in eight trained men riding a cycle ergometer at 4,300 m, but not at sea level. This positive effect was present after 1 hour of altitude exposure and tended to remain even after 2 weeks of acclimatization.

There is some debate about whether caffeine enhances cognitive performance or simply restores degraded psychomotor performance in rested individuals. The majority of studies that have examined the effects of caffeine in rested subjects studied moderate caffeine consumers (200–300 mg of caffeine per day) who were required to abstain from caffeine for some period of time prior to cognitive testing. Some researchers have speculated that for regular caffeine users, this abstinence could have resulted in some degree of withdrawal. Thus, beneficial effects on cognitive behavior may represent remediation of deteriorated performance during caffeine withdrawal back to baseline performance in the presence of caffeine rather than a net enhancement of performance.

A number of studies have demonstrated that caffeine enhances cognitive performance independent of its ability to reverse symptoms of withdrawal (see Chapter 3). Caffeine can enhance performance on some types of cognitive tasks and some aspects of mood in nonsleep-deprived individuals. Caffeine enhanced accuracy and reduced reaction time on auditory and visual vigilance tasks in a dose-related manner. Moreover, caffeine significantly increased self-reports of vigor and decreased reports of fatigue, depression, and hostility on the Profile of Moods Scale. Self-assessments of energy levels were also improved by caffeine. In a simulated military situation involving a tedious task that required sustained attention for proficient performance (i.e., sentry duty), caffeine eliminated the vigilance decrement that occurred with increasing time on duty, reduced subjective reports of tiredness, and did not impair rifle firing accuracy. Additionally, in this situation, caffeine increased the number of correct target identifications in both males and females.

Military personnel face many situations in which extended wakefulness may be required including sentry duty, deployment-related activities, air transportation during emergencies, radar and sonar monitoring, submarine duty, and combat. As part of their duties in these situations, individuals are required to perform complex cognitive tasks. The performance of these tasks is compromised during periods of extended wakefulness.

A variety of instruments have been used to quantify the effects of sleep deprivation on behavior. Alertness has been assessed using objective measures such as ambulatory vigilance monitors, visual and auditory vigilance tasks, and subjective measures such as self-reports and questionnaires. Studies using these measures have found that sleep deprivation impairs performance on vigilance tasks and decreases self-reports of alertness. A number of mental tasks, including mental arithmetic tasks, such as a serial add–subtract test, logical reasoning, mental rotation, perceptual cueing, and memory tests have been used to assess the effects of sleep deprivation on higher cognitive processes. Using these tests, mental performance deteriorates as a function of length of sleep deprivation.

All of the above-listed decrements in cognitive behavior can best be reversed by sleep. Any amount of sleep from as little as a 15-minute nap can restore some degree of function, although the longer the sleep episode, the greater the amount of cognitive function restored. Naps are effective both prior to (prophylactic naps) and during (restorative naps) a period of sleep deprivation. The only negative side effect of sleep in this context is sleep inertia, a period of mental confusion upon awakening from such naps that may last up to 30 minutes.

In sleep-deprived subjects, judicious use of caffeine can restore alertness, performance on mental tasks, and positive mood states. Caffeine reversed the sleep deprivation-induced increased response time, and increased alertness and performance on a visual vigilance task, mental arithmetic tests, and logical reasoning in sleep-deprived subjects. Caffeine is also effective in delaying sleep onset in sleep-deprived subjects. Using visual analog scales, caffeine intake led to reports of decreased sleepiness and increased alertness, ability to concentrate, confidence, talkativeness, energy levels, anxiety, jitteriness, and nervousness.

Conclusions

Caffeine at levels ranging from 200 to 600 mg/d enhances endurance performance in a variety of activities. Limited research has shown caffeine to be especially useful in restoring decrements in physical performance that occur at high altitudes. Food and fluid intake have to be monitored carefully when caffeine is used for this purpose, particularly at high altitudes and in hot environments. The documented declines in food intake during special operations would be of particular concern if food is the delivery vehicle chosen for administering caffeine.

Although there is considerable variation in doses tested and subject responses to the effects of caffeine on cognitive function, overall research shows that caffeine in the range of 100 to 600 mg is effective in increasing speed of reaction time without affecting accuracy and in improving performance on visual and audio vigilance tasks. A number of studies have also reported improved performance on long-term memory recall, but not short-term word recall. These enhancing effects of caffeine on cognitive performance are most pronounced when functions are impaired or suboptimal (e.g., as a result of sleep deprivation).

Recommendations

Caffeine in doses of 100 to 600 mg may be used to maintain cognitive performance, particularly in situations of sleep deprivation. Specifically, it can be used in maintaining speed of reactions and visual and auditory vigilance, which in military operations could be a life or death situation.

A similar dose range (200–600 mg) is also effective in enhancing physical endurance and may be especially useful in returning some of the physical function lost at high altitude. However, if caffeine is used either at high altitudes or in extremely hot environments, fluid and food intake of personnel should be monitored to ensure adequate intake.

2. **Safety: What are the medical risks to individuals associated with ready availability of caffeine, including acute health risks, long-term health risks, potential interaction with other drugs or factors specific to military operations, and potential problems of habituation of use?**

The effect of caffeine on various aspects of health has been and continues to be an active area of scientific research, in spite of the fact that caffeine has been used for more than 1,000 years without apparent ill effects. Over the past 100 years, the list of diseases in which caffeine has been implicated has changed. Convincing research evidence has removed several diseases from consideration, including various cancers, hypercholesteremia, and benign breast disease. Extensive research also has evaluated the impact of caffeine consumption on the incidence of hypertension, cardiovascular disease, reproduction and pregnancy outcome, osteoporosis, and fluid homeostasis. It has been shown that ingestion of very high doses of caffeine can produce undesirable effects on mental function. Additionally, caffeine use has been associated with physical dependence, which may be reflected in performance decrements during withdrawal under some circumstances.

Hypertension

Results summarized in recent reviews by Myers (in press) and Green and Suls (1996) suggest that caffeine-naive individuals may experience a small increase in blood pressure after acute dosing with caffeine. During chronic administration of caffeine, tolerance appears to develop, and chronic, long-lasting changes in blood pressure are usually not seen in individuals who consume caffeine routinely. A recent critical review of 30 years of controlled clinical and epidemiological studies on the blood pressure effects of coffee and caffeine (Nurminen et al., 1999) concluded that the acute pressor effects of caffeine are well documented, but that at present there is no clear epidemiological evidence that caffeine consumption is causally related to hypertension. They also concluded, however, that high caffeine intake may be an additional risk factor for hypertension at the individual level due to long-lasting stress or to a genetic susceptibility to hypertension.

Caffeine consumption has also been demonstrated to potentiate the effects of acute exercise and mental stress in increasing blood pressure. This effect of caffeine is more pronounced in those with high stress reactivity (i.e., high levels of anxiety) and those who are borderline hypertensive or are hypertensive.

Cardiovascular Disease

In spite of numerous studies (including controlled clinical trials) attempting to show a relationship between caffeine and serum lipoproteins, blood pressure, cardiac arrhythmias, and risk of coronary heart disease, results have failed to show a consistent adverse effect of ingestion of moderate amounts of caffeine. Whereas case-control studies have produced variable results, a meta-analysis of 11 prospective, longitudinal cohort studies showed no increased risk of coronary heart disease associated with consumption of up to 6 cups of coffee per day. Thus, increased risk of cardiovascular problems resulting from the use of caffeine supplements by the military would not appear to be of major concern in most cases.

Reproduction

Caffeine consumption has also been suggested as the cause of numerous negative reproductive outcomes, from shortened menstrual cycles to reduced conception, delayed implantation, spontaneous abortion, premature birth, low birthweight, and congenital malformations. As with most other aspects of caffeine consumption, there is a paucity of reliable data concerning the effects of caffeine on reproductive processes.

More recent reviews of human studies suggest that some of the initial reported associations between caffeine and reduced fertility, teratogenicity, and other fetal and maternal effects in humans may be explained by confounders such as associated cigarette smoking, alcohol consumption, reporting inaccuracies, and other methodological errors.

A recent well-controlled study of 487 women with spontaneous abortions and 2,087 normal controls, in which caffeine exposure was quantitated objectively by serum paraxanthine levels, showed that the mean serum paraxanthine concentration was significantly higher in women who had spontaneous abortions than in controls (752 versus 583 ng/mL). However, the odds ratio for spontaneous abortion was not significantly increased except in subjects with extremely high paraxanthine levels (> 1,845 ng/mL). These authors concluded that moderate consumption of caffeine was not likely to increase the risk of spontaneous abortion.

Osteoporosis

Caffeine consumption has been proposed as a risk factor for osteoporosis. The original observations stimulated several epidemiological studies that examined the possible relationship among caffeine consumption, calcium intake, and various indices of bone health. There appears to be no consistent trend linking caffeine consumption and negative effects on bone mineral density or incidence of fracture.

Although early experimental studies also indicated a significant effect on acute calcium diuresis, subsequent work indicated that this acute phase of excretion was accompanied by a later decrease in excretion of calcium in the urine. Moreover, later studies found either no significant effect of caffeine on calcium balance or negative balance only in subjects consuming less than about 660 mg of calcium per day, or half of the currently recommended intake of calcium.

Fluid Homeostasis

Consumption of 2,500 mL of a carbohydrate–electrolyte solution containing approximately 1 mg of caffeine per kg body weight increased 3-hour urine output by over 400 mL as compared to the same amount of solution without caffeine (Wemple et al., 1997). While this level of caffeine was too low to produce a positive effect on cycling performance, the fact that urine volume was affected could be of significance in military situations where considerably higher caffeine doses may be used. An oral dose of 250 mg of caffeine increased diuresis, sodium, potassium, and osmol excretion within 1 hour post-treatment (Nussberger et al., 1990), while amounts of coffee sufficient to provide 642 mg of caffeine in a single day caused a highly significant increase in 24-hour urine output of 753 ± 532 mL compared to an identical amount of fluid provided as mineral water. Total body water as measured by bioelectrical impedance decreased 2.7 percent, and sodium and potassium excretion increased by 66 and 28 percent, respectively (Neuhauser-Berthold et al., 1997). The information to date is inconsistent, indicating that caffeine may or may not create a total body water deficit. The deficit may depend on the amount of caffeine consumed, the individual's history of caffeine use, and the total solute load of any accompanying food or beverage. However, the risk of water deficit may be increased when caffeine is used in situations already known to put personnel at risk of dehydration, such as in hot or desert environments (IOM, 1993), or in cold environments (IOM, 1996).

Behavioral Effects

One potential risk of high doses of caffeine, which needs further substantiation, is dose-related decrements in mental functioning. A number of researchers have found that high doses of caffeine can adversely affect mental performance. Although a relatively low dose of caffeine (250 mg) produced favorable subjective effects (e.g., elation, pleasantness) and enhanced performance on cognitive tasks in healthy volunteers, higher doses (500 mg) led to less favorable subjective reports (e.g., tension, nervousness, anxiety, restlessness) and less improvement in cognitive performance than placebo. Negative effects may be more pronounced in nonusers than in regular users of caffeine. Caffeine has been shown to produce anxiety or panic attacks in individuals with agoraphobia or panic disorders, but not in healthy controls. However, caffeine has been shown to potentiate hormonal responses to other stressors.

Physical Dependence and Withdrawal

The use of caffeine by humans is generally not associated with abuse or addiction. Tolerance develops to some of the physiological effects of caffeine when caffeine-containing beverages are consumed regularly; however, there have been no reports of tolerance for caffeine effects on cognitive performance. Withdrawal symptoms can occur with the abrupt removal of caffeine from the diet. The symptoms of cessation, when they do occur, are not long-lasting and are generally mild. These include headaches, drowsiness, irritability, fatigue, low vigor, and flu-like symptoms.

Caffeine acts as a vasoconstrictor of the cerebral arteries, reducing regional blood flow. Caffeine withdrawal also causes changes in cerebral blood flow, resulting in vasodilation in persons with high caffeine intake that is thought to be associated with a throbbing, vascular-type headache, one of the most commonly observed symptoms of caffeine withdrawal. This withdrawal phenomenon could conceivably lead to decrements in performance during military operations.

Caffeine and Stress

Among the variables that may contribute to differences in caffeine sensitivity are baseline levels of stress exposure and genetically mediated stress reactivity. Stress may include physical stress (e.g., exercise), physiological stress (e.g., heat stress, infection, sleep deprivation), or psychological stress. After stress exposures, stress-responsive neurohormonal and neurotransmitter systems are activated, with associated release of the stress hormones and the adrenergic neurotransmitters (epinephrine, norepinephrine, corteotrophin-releasing hormone, adrenocorticotropic hormone, and cortisol), which all interact with caffeine. Caffeine alters the degree of responsiveness of these systems to stressful stimuli. For example, caffeine has been shown to increase plasma norepinephrine and to potentiate epinephrine and cortisol stress-reactivity to acute psychosocial stress. The degree of responsiveness in these studies varied according to previous caffeine consumption (habitual users versus nonusers).

Conclusions

The acute pressor effects of caffeine are well documented, but at present there is no clear epidemiological evidence that caffeine consumption is causally related to hypertension. One potential risk should be noted, however. A number of studies have demonstrated that caffeine consumption produces a transient elevation in blood pressure and that this occurs regardless of whether or not the individual is a habitual user of caffeine. In borderline-hypertensive men, the use of caffeine in situations of behavioral stress may elevate blood pressure to a clinically meaningful degree; it has been hypothesized that these types of blood pressure increases in hypertensives would be large enough to transiently reduce the therapeutic effects of antihypertensive medication. However, other studies have found no differences in the effect of caffeine in individuals with or without a family history of hypertension, and no difference in 24-hour ambulatory blood pressure in treated hypertensives between caffeinated and decaffeinated coffee. Thus, high caffeine intake may be an additional risk factor for hypertension at the individual level due to long-lasting stress or to a genetic susceptibility to hypertension. Since military scenarios in which the use of caffeine supplements might be desirable would frequently occur when personnel are also under acute mental and/or physical stress, this could be a concern to those personnel with family histories of hypertension.

In spite of numerous studies attempting to show a relationship between caffeine and cardiovascular health, results have failed to show a consistent adverse effect of ingestion of moderate amounts of caffeine. Increased risk of coronary heart disease resulting from the use of caffeine supplements by the military would not appear to be of major concern.

Results of studies of the effects of caffeine on reproduction have been very mixed, and many of those showing increased reproductive problems have been confounded with other life-style factors, particularly smoking. The most convincing evidence relates to caffeine and the increased risk of spontaneous abortion. However, since this requires caffeine consumption during the first trimester of pregnancy, it is likely to be a concern for sustained military operations only if female personnel are unaware of their pregnancy at the time of deployment.

The preponderance of research on caffeine and osteoporosis has found no relationship. Although caffeine can increase calcium diuresis, this is compensated by subsequent lower than normal calcium excretion. The use of caffeine in this case is less of a concern than is low calcium intake.

Caffeine functions as a diuretic, and this effect appears to increase with increasing caffeine level. Evidence is equivocal as to whether acute doses of caffeine cause a total body water deficit. The increased risk of dehydration may be of concern for military personnel in operational environments where dehydration may already be a concern, such as desert environments, or where thirst mechanisms are inadequate, such as in cold or high-altitude environments.

High doses of caffeine (> 600 mg) can cause decrements in cognitive function. Negative effects may be more pronounced in nonusers than in regular users of caffeine. Caffeine can also potentiate the effects of stress.

Recommendations

Use of caffeine under conditions of sustained operations (SUSOPS) would not appear to pose any acute or chronic health risks for military personnel.

Caffeine use in SUSOPS in hot environments, cold environments, or at high altitudes may increase the risk of dehydration, and fluid and food intake of personnel should be closely monitored in these situations.

Female military personnel should be advised of the potential for a slight increase in risk of spontaneous abortion in the first trimester of pregnancy.

3. Dose and Warning Labels: What dose level should be recommended to habituated caffeine users and to nonusers? What warnings should be provided on such a product in the context of ethical, religious, and potential caffeine habituation concerns?

The effective doses of caffeine will vary from individual to individual depending on a variety of factors including time of day, usual caffeine intake, and whether the individual is rested, smokes, or uses oral contraceptives. Doses evaluated experimentally for their effects on both physical and cognitive performance have ranged from as little as 32 mg of caffeine (Lieberman et al., 1987) to as much as 1,400 mg (Streufert et al., 1997).

The levels of caffeine that have consistently enhanced endurance performance, as discussed in Chapter 3, range from about 150 to 600 mg. Numerous studies of the effects of different caffeine dosages on various aspects of cognitive performance have been conducted in both civilian and military situations. Levels of caffeine in the range of 100 to 400 mg have consistently demonstrated reductions in reaction time and enhanced performance on vigilance tests, whereas levels of caffeine in excess of 600 mg have shown negative effects on mood and behavior (negative effects may be seen at lower levels in individuals nonhabituated to caffeine).

In sleep-deprived individuals (similar to those engaging in SUSOPS), levels in the range of 100 to 600 mg of caffeine appear to improve performance (e.g., vigilance, mood, higher cognitive functions) with few acute adverse behavioral effects; some of the positive effects persist for 8–10 hours. Even individuals who do not normally consume caffeine appear to obtain these caffeine-related positive effects.

Important ethical considerations include providing personnel with adequate information and training on the use of the product, providing the opportunity for personnel to test the product in a nonoperational situation, and use of a product that allows individual control of the dosage.

Regular moderate to heavy users of caffeine may experience headaches, fatigue, and drowsiness if denied access to caffeine.

Conclusions

A caffeine dose of 100–600 mg can be expected to improve vigilance and enhance cognitive performance regardless of an individual's normal caffeine status. A delivery mechanism that provides 100-mg dose increments could be used to allow individuals of smaller body size, nonhabituated caffeine users, and those with heightened sensitivity to caffeine to individually control their dose.

In keeping with the rulings of the U.S. Food and Drug Administration (FDA) with respect to determination of the risks of caffeine as a food additive, no warning label is necessary for a military product designed for maintenance of cognitive performance during sustained operations. However, educational and training information is needed for military personnel prior to the use of such a product.

Recommendations

A caffeine delivery vehicle that provides caffeine in 100-mg increments with a total content not exceeding approximately 600 mg would appear to be the most appropriate dose for use in sustained military operations. Since there is little information regarding the extent to which tolerance to caffeine's cognitive effects in habitual users develops, no differential dosing is recommended for habitual compared to first-time caffeine users. For subsequent dosing, the dosing interval should be based on the considerations that too-frequent dosing might (1) produce a buildup of caffeine (or its primary metabolite, paraxanthine) levels sufficient to precipitate negative effects; and (2) inhibit sleep onset in some individuals at a time when sleep is desired. Since the half-life of caffeine in blood can vary from 1.5 to 9.5 hours, with an average half-life of 4 to 5 hours, a dosing interval of no less than 3 to 4 hours is recommended.

Any product that is used as a vehicle for providing caffeine to military personnel should be prominently labeled. The labeling should include a statement on the principal display panel that the product contains added caffeine and should only be used to maintain performance when involved in SUSOPS or sustained vigilance activities. The message on the principal display panel should direct the user to specific information elsewhere on the label that indicates the level of caffeine per unit of product and the total amount per package or container. An example is shown in Box 7-1. This content information is vital for the command structure to make decisions about directions for use and for individuals to adapt consumption to their individual needs.

An in-depth training program on the benefits, directions for use, and potential side effects or symptoms of excess intake of caffeine should be designed for command personnel. In addition, if caffeine is to be used to enhance performance, military personnel should be given adequate training to ensure the benefits of caffeine supplementation and avoid any potential side effects. Such training should include the use of caffeine during periods of sleep deprivation and possibly altered work–rest cycles. All personnel should test the effects of the recommended dose in a nonoperational situation prior to use in an operational situation.

> **BOX 7-1** Example of an information statement for a caffeine-containing supplement.
>
> ! IMPORTANT !
> This product contains 100 mg of added caffeine per unit (e.g., 1 pill, 1 food bar segment, 1 stick of gum) for a total added caffeine content of 600 mg, and is designed for use in maintaining alertness during military operations. Recommended initial dose is 200 mg.
> Do not exceed 600 mg in a single dose.
> Do not repeat dose sooner than 3–4 hours.

Military personnel who regularly consume caffeine-containing products should not be denied access to these products in anticipation of the use of a caffeine supplement. Symptoms of withdrawal such as fatigue, decreased alertness, and headaches could cause decrements in performance prior to the consumption of the caffeine supplement.

4. Alternatives: Are there practical alternatives to caffeine that would better serve the intended purpose of enhancing or maintaining performance in fatigued service members?

Sleep is the most effective means of reconstituting the decrements in cognitive functioning brought on by sleep deprivation. Thus, in situations where it is feasible, sleep should be promoted. There is a dose effect for the restorative effects of sleep duration on cognitive performance (Bonnet, 1999; Bonnet and Arand, 1994a,b; Bonnet et al., 1995; Dinges et al., 1987). Any amount of sleep from as little as a 15-minute nap can restore some degree of function, although the longer the sleep episode, the greater the amount of cognitive function restored (Bonnet et al., 1995). Dinges et al. (1987) demonstrated that prophylactic naps were better than restorative naps and were more important than circadian placement of naps.

Combination of Caffeine and Naps

The most effective nonprescription drug alternative to caffeine administration alone when a normal sleep regimen is not possible, is a combination of caffeine and naps. The combination of caffeine and naps increased alertness during long periods of sleep deprivation compared to either caffeine or naps alone. The committee recommends that wherever possible, commanders adopt strategies that incorporate the use of caffeine with short naps for maintaining vigilance, alertness, and other physiological and cognitive functions needed for SUSOPS. According to the literature reviewed in this report, naps taken early in the period of extended wakefulness followed by caffeine taken around the time of circadian troughs would be most effective.

Amphetamine

In extensive simulator and in-flight testing, amphetamine was observed by investigators (Caldwell and Caldwell, 1997; Caldwell et al., 1995) to "improve subjective feelings of fatigue, confusion, and depression while increasing feelings of vigor". Amphetamine is, however, a controlled substance and thus requires an individual medical evaluation to determine risk factors and health status before a prescription can be issued. With appropriate supervision and control, the use of amphetamine has benefited individuals with unique skills whose performance was critical to the safety of personnel and complex military hardware. In contrast to caffeine in food, beverages, chewing gum, and pill or tablet form, there is little experience with amphetamine pill self-dosing for most military personnel, and the hazards and adverse effects of self-dosing might therefore be expected to be greater. It would be preferable if ergogenic effects can be achieved without such substances. The potential for abuse of amphetamines is considerable, and the appropriate monitoring of its dispensing and use may add unnecessary burdens to medical personnel in the intense and demanding tasks that are directly involved in guaranteeing the success of SUSOPS. Although amphetamine (20 mg) was effective in reversing the negative effects on alertness during sleep deprivation and these effects are greater than those of caffeine at 300 mg, it had deleterious effects on recovery sleep, which also may be important in the ultimate success of demanding and constantly changing SUSOPS (Bray et al., 1999). Amphetamine should not be considered as a substitute for sleep, and more nights of recovery sleep may be needed after its administration (Caldwell, 1999). Therefore, considerable caution is warranted, and use of this stimulant should be restricted to only the most extreme circumstances when such measures are considered essential to the success of highly sensitive operations. Clearly, more research should be done before consideration can be given to the routine use of amphetamine.

Modafinil

Modafinil is a new prescription drug approved by the FDA as a wakefulness-promoting substance. It has undergone evaluation as a treatment for excessive daytime sleepiness (EDS) in narcolepsy (Broughton et al., 1997). This drug appears to be useful in reducing EDS without effecting voluntary nap or nocturnal sleep initiation. These properties suggest that the stimulant may be useful in extending high levels of vigilance in SUSOPS. A number of studies have examined the effects of modafinil on cognitive performance and sleep recovery in sleep-deprived, but otherwise healthy, volunteers. Modafinil (300 mg) was as effective as 20 mg of dextroamphetamine in maintaining both subjective estimates of mood and fatigue, and objective measures of cognitive performance when administered three times during 64 hours of sleep deprivation (Pigeau et al., 1995), with no effects on recovery sleep (Buguet et al., 1995). Another study compared the effects of 300 mg of modafinil every 24 hours to placebo in healthy individuals during 60 hours of sleep deprivation using the visual search paradigm for assessing speed and accuracy in target detection. Slow search rates and number of errors increased linearly in the placebo condition with increasing time without sleep, but remained the same as rested controls with modafinil (Stivalet et al., 1998). Batejat and Lagarde (1999) examined the effects of 200 mg of modafinil in conjunction with naps on performance during two 27-hour periods of sleep deprivation. Modafinil maintained an efficient level of central nervous system (CNS) general activation close to awakening. As in previous studies, modafinil did not prevent sleep if sleep opportunities were available.

Caldwell et al. (1999) recently reported on the use of modafinil in a helicopter simulator study with pilots exposed to two 40-hour periods of sleep deprivation. Three 200-mg doses of modafinil or placebo were administered during the 40-hour period. Modafinil significantly attenuated the effects of sleep deprivation on four of six flight maneuvers, reduced the amount of slow-wave electroencephalogram activity (indicative of reduced CNS activation), lessened self-reported problems with mood and alertness, and curtailed the performance decrements that were found with placebo. The most noticeable benefit of the drug was seen when the combined impact of sleep loss and circadian trough was most severe.

Conclusions

Providing the opportunity and environment for adequate sleep is the ideal but is obviously impractical for continuous military operations. Combining naps with judicious caffeine use may be the best remedy for sleep deprivation-induced decrements in cognitive function in military situations where adequate sleep cannot be obtained. When naps are not an option, caffeine alone could be used to mitigate sleep deprivation-induced impairments in cognitive behavior for up to 24 hours of sleep deprivation.

The Department of Defense (DOD) has precedents for the use of prescription drugs in healthy individuals, such as the use of amphetamines. Furthermore, in the United States, physicians are permitted to prescribe drugs for off-label use (i.e., for uses not included in the product's labeling).

The use of amphetamine is superior to caffeine in offsetting decrements in cognitive performance; however, the risks outweigh the benefits for most situations. It is a controlled substance, it has a high abuse potential, and it interferes with recovery sleep. In addition, it is assumed that the majority of combat personnel would not have had previous experience with the drug.

The drug modafanil, which was developed more than 10 years ago as a treatment for narcolepsy, shows considerable promise. It appears to be as effective as amphetamines in offsetting performance degradation, does not interfere with recovery sleep, is not an appetite suppressant, and appears to have a much lower abuse potential.

Recommendations

It is recommended that the military have in place a doctrine related to the importance of sleep prior to extended missions and the importance of naps whenever possible during operations. Naps would be most effective when taken early in the period of sleep deprivation. Of the psychostimulant compounds, caffeine would be the compound of choice, since many personnel would have personal experience with the compound, it is not a restricted substance, it does not interfere with recovery sleep following periods of sleep deprivation, and it is generally considered to have very low abuse potential.

The DOD should continue to research the drug modafinil to further explore its potential for sustaining cognitive performance during military operations. Research published to date indicates that it may prove far superior to caffeine in maintaining cognitive performance over extended periods of sleep deprivation, without the adverse side effects and abuse potential of amphetamines.

5. Formulation: (a) Does the inclusion of other components (e.g., glucose) improve the beneficial effects of caffeine in sustained operations, as previously suggested by the committee? (b) Is there a better approach to caffeine delivery than the nutrient bar currently produced for the military?

The evidence is unclear on the utility of adding glucose or other carbohydrates to caffeine to further enhance physical performance. Caffeine enhances the availability of free fatty acids and decreases glycogenolysis, whereas carbohydrate as glucose increases the availability, and presumably the use, of this substrate. Some researchers have proposed that caffeine be delivered in a carbohydrate-containing medium to further enhance performance. However, most studies to date have been flawed in some way and reported variable results. Additional well-designed research is still necessary regarding the combined effects of caffeine and carbohydrate on physical performance. No studies were found in the published literature that examined the effects of caffeine combined with other nutrients on cognitive performance, and this may be an area for further research.

There may be nutritional reasons (e.g., provision of food energy, nutrients, or fluid) for including caffeine in a food form. A chocolate bar has been formulated by the military and found to be acceptable in preference studies. The bars have also been used as delivery vehicles for other food constituents such as tyrosine, creatine, and antioxidant nutrients that might enhance performance under certain circumstances.

The committee considered various approaches to caffeine delivery for SUSOPS, including the food/energy bar and other alternatives such as caffeinated chewing gum, tablets (both sustained release and regular), and beverages. In assessing the alternatives, the pros and cons of each of these vehicles were considered. Their major characteristics are summarized in Table 7-1. There is good evidence that caffeine is absorbed rapidly and completely from the gut when supplied in a liquid form, with virtually all (99 percent) of the administered dose absorbed in about 45 minutes (Blanchard and Sawers, 1983; Chvasta and Cooke, 1971). However, the committee is unaware of evidence on the absorption of caffeine from a food matrix, as in solid foods such as bars. Theoretically, absorption should be slower than it is from liquids because gastric emptying time might be slower. Lipid solubility and possibly caffeine absorption in the stomach may influence these processes as well. Studies of the rapidity of absorption and action of caffeine are needed for such bars if they are to be considered as a caffeine delivery vehicle.

A caffeine delivery vehicle that is most appropriate in one setting may not be so in another, as presented in Table 7-1. Caffeine in a food matrix may be advantageous when it is important to deliver nutrients, fluid, or other food constituents simultaneously, but the satiating effects of the food may somewhat limit consumption, especially if high intakes are required to obtain a sufficient dose. Chewing gums are more appropriate if rapid absorption and action are needed, and would facilitate tailoring of individual doses. Caffeine in a fluid or gel matrix may be more appropriate when dehydration is an issue.

Various characteristics of the individual also alter the effects of a given dose of caffeine. These involve both individual factors (e.g., age, sex, smoker versus nonsmoker) and states that can vary greatly from one situation to another (e.g., stress hormonal status, ingestion of certain drugs, illness, heat stress, sleep status); thus, the delivered dose may have different psychological and physiological effects at one time than it does at another.

Conclusions

A summary of the characteristics of different methods of caffeine delivery is presented in Table 7-1. Although evidence of a potentiating effect of carbohydrates on caffeine effectiveness is equivocal, there are other reasons to consider providing supplemental nutrients along with the caffeine. For example, inadequate food and fluid intake is a common problem during military operations. The use of a caffeinated chewing gum would appear to provide the most rapid absorption.

TABLE 7-1 Summary of Potential Caffeine Delivery Approaches

Vehicle	Dose of Caffeine	Other Components That Improve Beneficial Effects of Caffeine?	Weight or Volume
Food bar	600 mg caffeine, scored in 150-mg increments	Yes—sucrose and corn syrup are simple sugars that may enhance the positive effects of caffeine on certain aspects of physical performance (depending on the type of exercise being performed); also contains complex carbohydrate, fat, and protein	70 g
Food bar, modified dose	100 mg increments	Yes—sucrose and corn syrup are simple sugars that may enhance the positive effects of caffeine on certain aspects of physical performance (depending on the type of exercise being performed); also contains complex carbohydrate, fat, and protein	50 g
Caffeinated soft drinks	Caffeine content varies from 5 to 50 mg depending on type and source	Yes—Sucrose and corn syrup are present in regular brands, aspartame in diet brands	12 fluid oz (36 g)
Caffeinated chewing gum	100 mg/stick	Yes—sucrose, corn syrup; also contains small amounts of glycerin, lecithin, and aspartame	? 5 g
Caffeine pills	100 mg	No	—
Sustained release caffeine	200 or 300 mg	No	—

Possible Rapidity of Absorption	Likely Rapidity of Action	Abuse Potential	Comments
? Slower	? Slower	Low	Bioavailability uncertain; good vehicle for providing other nutrients or food constituents such as sugars if these prove to be useful; more bulky than chewing gum or pills; satiating effects possible if caffeine content is low
? Slower	? Slower	Low	Bioavailability uncertain; good vehicle for providing other nutrients or food constituents such as sugars; satiating effects possible if caffeine content low; more bulky than chewing gum or pills
Rapid (< 60 min)	Rapid	Low	Provide fluid; good vehicle for sugars if these prove useful; more bulky than chewing gum or pills; a dehydrated beverage powder requires water and time to mix
Most rapid	Most rapid	Low	Absorbed sublingually and rapidly; low bulk; no or little satiating effects likely
Rapid	Rapid	Low	Bioavailability somewhat lower than from caffeinated drinks; no satiating effects likely
Initial dose rapid, sustained release	Initially rapid followed by slower absorption	Low	Permits longer intervals between doses but less flexibility during suddenly altered operational situations

Environmental circumstances and individual characteristics may make one caffeine delivery vehicle appropriate in some circumstances and inappropriate in another.

Recommendations

If food/energy bars are used, they must be tested for the rapidity of caffeine absorption and action. Under certain circumstances such as heat stress or desert operations, chewing gums may offer practical operational advantages over a food/energy bar, but under other conditions, such as reconnaissance operations from a central point, the bar may be preferable. Thus, more than one delivery vehicle should be considered, provided complete data on absorption and rapidity of action are available. In terms of convenience, pills or capsules could be considered, however, the little data available suggest that the bioavailability of caffeine in this form is less than in oral liquids. In addition, the use of pills or capsules does not meet the Army's stated preference of providing performance aids in the context of a food or beverage.

ADDITIONAL RESEARCH RECOMMENDATIONS

In reviewing the caffeine literature for this report, it became clear that there are still gaps in the knowledge database concerning caffeine and other potential cognitive enhancers that may be of military relevance. These are:

- bioavailability of caffeine from substances other than liquids consumed orally;
- additional research on the effectiveness and optimal doses of the wakefulness-promoting drug, modafinil, in simulated combat environments;
- effectiveness of various combinations of naps and caffeine;
- effects of consumption of greater than recommended doses of caffeine on fluid homeostasis in different environments (e.g., consumption of the total 600 mg caffeine delivery product in a hot, cold, or high-altitude environment); and
- properly designed studies on the effects of caffeine combined with other nutrients (e.g., carbohydrate, fat) on physical and cognitive performance.

References

Abernethy DR, Todd EL. 1985. Impairment of caffeine clearance by chronic use of low-dose estrogen-containing oral contraceptives. *Eur J Clin Pharmacol* 28:425–428.

Acquaviva F, DeFrancesco A, Adnruilli A, Piantino P, Arrigoni A, Massarenti P, Balzola F. 1986. Effect of regular and decaffeinated coffee on serum gastrin levels. *J Clin Gastroenterol* 8:150–153.

Akerstedt T, Ficca G. 1997. Alertness-enhancing drugs as a countermeasure to fatigue in irregular work hours. *Chronobiol Int* 14:145–158.

Amendola CA, Gabrieli JDE, Lieberman HR. 1998. Caffeine's effects on performance and mood are independent of age and gender. *Nutr Neurosci* 1:269–280.

Angrist B, Corwin J, Bartlik B, Cooper T. 1987. Early pharmacokinetics and clinical effects of oral D-amphetamine in normal subjects. *Biol Psychiatry* 22:1357–1368.

Anonymous. 1992a. Amphetamines. In: *Drug Facts and Comparisons.* St. Louis: Wolters Kluwer Co. Pp. 1022–1026.

Anonymous. 1992b. Pemoline. In: *Drug Facts and Comparisons.* St. Louis: Wolters Kluwer Co. Pp. 1301–1302.

Anselme F, Collomp K, Mercier B, Ahmaidi S, Prefaut C. 1992. Caffeine increases maximal anaerobic power and blood lactate concentration. *Eur J Appl Physiol* 65:188–191.

Arciero PJ, Gardner AW, Calles-Escandon J, Benowitz NL, Poehlman ET. 1995. Effects of caffeine ingestion on NE kinetics, fat oxidation, and energy expenditure in younger and older men. *Am J Physiol* 268:E1192–E1198.

Arciero PJ, Gardner AW, Benowitz NL, Poehlman ET. 1998. Relationship of blood pressure, heart rate and behavioral mood state to norepinephrine kinetics in younger and older men following caffeine ingestion. *Eur J Clin Nutr* 52:805–812.

Armstrong LE, Maresh CM. 1996. Fluid replacement during exercise and recovery from exercise. In: Buskirk ER, Puhl SM, eds. *Body Fluid Balance: Exercise and Sport.* Boca Raton, FL: CRC Press. Pp. 259–282.

Arnaud MJ. 1987. The pharmacology of caffeine. *Prog Drug Res* 31: 273–313.

Arnaud MJ. 1988. The metabolism of coffee constituents. In: Coffee. Volume 3: Physiology. pp. 33–55.

Arnaud MJ. 1993. Metabolism of caffeine and other components of coffee. In: Garattini S, ed. Caffeine, Coffee, and Health. New York: Raven Press. Pp. 43–95.

Babkoff H, Kelly TL, Matteson LT, Gomez S, Lopez A, Hauser S, Naitoh P. 1992. Pemoline and methylphenidate: Interaction with mood, sleepiness, and cognitive performance during 64 hours of sleep deprivation. Mil Psychol 4:235–265.

Bak AA, Grobbee DE. 1991. Caffeine, blood pressure, and serum lipids. Am J Clin Nutr 53:971–975.

Balogh A, Irmisch E, Klinger G, Splinter FK, Hoffmann A. 1987. Elimination of caffeine and metamizol in the menstrual cycle of the fertile female. Zent bl Gyndkol 109:1135–1142.

Barger-Lux MJ, Heaney RP, Stegman MR. 1990. Effects of moderate caffeine intake on the calcium economy of premenopausal women. Am J Clin Nutr 52:722–725.

Barone JJ, Roberts HH. 1996. Caffeine consumption. Food Chem Toxicol 34:119–129.

Batejat DM, Lagarde DP. 1999. Naps and modafinil as countermeasures for the effects of sleep deprivation on cognitive performance. Aviat Space Environ Med 70:493–498.

Bell DG, Jacobs I. 1999. Combined caffeine and ephedrine ingestion improves run times of Canadian Forces Warrior Test. Aviat Space Environ Med 70:325–329.

Bell DG, Jacobs I, McLellan TM, Miyazaki M, Sabiston CM. 1999. Thermal regulation in heat during exercise after caffeine and ephedrine ingestion. Aviat Space Environ Med 70:583–588.

Belland KM, Bissell C. 1994. A subjective study of fatigue during Navy flight operations over southern Iraq: Operation Southern Watch. Aviat Space Environ Med 65:557–561.

Benowitz NL. 1990. Clinical pharmacology of caffeine. Annu Rev Med 41:277–288.

Benowitz NL, Jacob P III, Mayan H, Denaro C. 1995. Sympathomimetic effects of paraxanthine and caffeine in humans. Clin Pharmacol Ther 58:684–691.

Berglund B, Hemmingsson P. 1982. Effects of caffeine ingestion on exercise performance at low and high altitudes in cross country skiers. Int J Sports Med 3:234–236.

Blanchard J, Sawers SJA. 1983. Comparative pharmacokinetics of caffeine in young and elderly men. J Pharmacokinet Biopharm 11:109–126.

Bonati M, Latini R, Galletti F, Young JF, Tognoni G, Garattini S. 1982. Caffeine disposition after oral doses. Clin Pharmacol Ther 32:98–106.

Bonnet MH. 1993. Cognitive effects of sleep and sleep fragmentation. Sleep 16:S65–S67.

Bonnet M. 1999. Use of Prophylactic Naps Versus Caffeine to Maintain Alertness During Periods of Sleep Loss. Presented at the Institute of Medicine Workshop on Caffeine Formulations for Sustainment of Mental Task Performance During Military Operations, Washington, DC, February 2–3. Committee on Military Nutrition Research.

Bonnet MH, Arand DL. 1994a. Impact of naps and caffeine on extended nocturnal performance. Physiol Behav 56:103–109.

Bonnet MH, Arand DL. 1994b. The use of prophylactic naps and caffeine to maintain performance during a continuous operation. Ergonomics 37:1009–1020.

Bonnet MH, Gomez S, Wirth O, Arand DL. 1995. The use of caffeine versus prophylactic naps in sustained performance. Sleep 18:97–104.

Boulenger JP, Uhde TW, Wolff EA III, Post RM. 1984. Increased sensitivity to caffeine in patients with panic disorders. Preliminary Evidence. Arch Gen Psychiatry 41:1067–1071.

REFERENCES

Brachtel D, Richter E. 1992. Absolute bioavailability of caffeine from a tablet formulation. J Hepatol 16:385.

Brackett LE, Daly TW. 1991. Relaxant effects of adenosine analogs on guinea pig trachea in vitro. Xanthine-sensitive and xanthine-insensitive mechanisms. J Pharmacol Exp Ther 257:205–213.

Brackett LE, Sharnim MT, Daly JW. 1990. Activities of caffeine, theophylline and enprofylline analogs as tracheal relaxants. Biochem Pharmacol 39:1897–1904.

Bray G, Lieberman H, Magill R, Ryan D, Smith S, Volaufova J, Waters W. 1999. Caffeine Effects During Sleep Deprivation and Recovery. Presented at the Institute of Medicine Workshop on Caffeine Formulations for Sustainment of Mental Task Performance During Military Operations, Washington, DC, February 2–3. Committee on Military Nutrition Research.

Broughton RJ, Fleming JAE, George CFP, Hill JD, Kryger MH, Moldofsky H, Montplaisir JY, Morehouse RL, Moscovitch A, Murphy WF. 1997. Randomized, double-blinded, placebo-controlled crossover trial of modafinil in the treatment of excessive daytime sleepiness in narcolepsy. Neurology 49:444–451.

Brouns F, Kovacs MR, Senden JMG. 1998. The effect of different rehydration drinks on post-exercise electrolyte excretion in trained athletes. Int J Sports Med 19:56–60.

Brown NJ, Ryder D, Nadeau J. 1993. Caffeine attenuates the renal vascular response to angiotensin II infusion. Hypertension 22:847–852.

Buguet A, Montmayeur A, Pigeau R, Naitoh P. 1995. Modafinil, d-amphetamine and placebo during 64 hours of sustained mental work. II. Effects on two nights of recovery sleep. J Sleep Res 4:229–241.

Burg AW, Werner E. 1975. Effect of orally administered caffeine and theophylline on the tissue concentrations of 3'5'-cyclic AMP and phosphodiesterase. Federation Proc 34: 332.

Busto U, Bendayan R, Sellers EM. 1989. Clinical pharmacokinetics of non-opiate abused drugs. Clin Pharmacokinet 16:1–26.

Caan B, Quesenberry CP Jr, Coates AP. 1998. Differences in fertility associated with caffeinated beverage consumption. Am J Public Health 88:270–274.

Caldwell J. 1999. Use of Amphetamines to Counteract Sleep Deprivation. Presented at the Institute of Medicine Workshop on Caffeine Formulations for Sustainment of Mental Task Performance During Military Operations, Washington, DC, February 2–3. Committee on Military Nutrition Research.

Caldwell JA, Caldwell JL. 1997. An in-flight investigation of the efficacy of dextroamphetamine for sustaining helicopter flight performance. *Aviat Space Environ Med* 68:1073–1080.

Caldwell JA, Caldwell JL, Crowley JS, Jones HD. 1995. Sustaining helicopter pilot performance with Dexadrine® during periods of sleep deprivation. *Aviat Space Environ Med* 66:930–937.

Caldwell JA, Nicholas K, Caldwell JL, Hall KK, Norman DN. 1999. *The Effects of Modafinil on Aviator Performance During 40 Hours of Continuous Wakefulness: A UH-60 Helicopter Simulator Study*. Report No. USAARL-99-17. Fort Rucker, AL: Army Aeromedical Research Unit.

Caldwell JA, Smythe NK, Leduc PA, Caldwell JL. 2000. Efficacy of Dexadrine® for maintaining aviator performance during 64 hours of sustained wakefulness: A simulator study. *Aviat Space Environ Med* 71:7–18.

Callahan MM, Robertson RS, Arnaud MJ, Branfman AR, McCormish MF, Yesair DW. 1982. Human metabolism of [1-*methyl*-^{14}C]- and [2-^{14}C]caffeine after oral administration. *Drug Metab Dispos* 10:417–423.

Cameron OG, Modell JG, Harihaven M. 1990. Caffeine and human cerebral blood flow: A positron emission tomography study. *Life Sci* 47:1141–1146.

Castellanos FX, Rapoport JL. In press. Effects of caffeine on development and behavior in infancy and childhood: A review of the Medline literature. In: *Caffeine and Health*. Washington, DC: ILSI North America.

Charney DS, Heninger GR, Jatlow PI. 1985. Increased anxiogenic effects of caffeine in panic disorders. *Arch Gen Psychiatry* 4293:233–243.

Chelsky LB, Cutler JE, Griffith K, Kron J, McClelland JH, and McAnulty JH. 1990. Caffeine and ventricular arrhythmias. An electrophysiological approach. *J Am Med Assoc* 264:2236–2240.

Chemelli RM, Willie JT, Sinton CM, Elmquist JK, Scammell T, Lee C, Richardson JA, Williams SC, Xiong Y, Kisanuko Y, Fitch TE, Nakazato M, Hammer RE, Saper CB, Yanagisawa M. 1999. Narcolepsy in orexin knockout mice: Molecular genetics of sleep regulation. *Cell* 98:437–451.

Christian MS, Brent RL. 2001. Teratogen update: Evaluation of the reproductive and developmental risks of caffeine. *Teratology* 64:51–78.

Chvasta TE, Cooke AR. 1971. Emptying and absorption of caffeine from the human stomach. *Gastroenterology* 61:838–843.

Cohen BS, Nelson AG, Prevost MC, Thompson GD, Marx BD, Morris GS. 1996. Effects of caffeine ingestion on endurance racing in the heat and humidity. *Eur J Appl Physiol* 73:358–363.

Collis MG, Keddie JR, Torr SR. 1984. Evidence that the positive ionotropic effects of alkylxanthines are not due to adenosine receptor blockade. *Br J Pharmacol* 81:401–407.

Collomp K, Ahmaidi S, Chatard JC, Audran M, Prefaut C. 1992. Benefits of caffeine ingestion on sprint performance in trained and untrained swimmers. *Eur J Appl Physiol* 64:377–380.

Couturier EG, Laman DM, van Duijn MA, van Duijn H. 1997. Influence of coffee and caffeine withdrawal on headache and cerebral blood flow velocities. *Cephalalgia* 17:188–190.

Curatolo PW, Robertson D. 1983. The health consequences of caffeine: Review. *Ann Intern Med* 98:641–653.

Daly JW. 1993. Mechanism of action of caffeine. In: Garattini S, ed. *Caffeine, Coffee, and Health*. New York: Raven Press. Pp. 97–150.

Daly JW, Shi D, Nikodyivic O, Jacobson KA. 1999. The role of adenosine receptors in the central action of caffeine. In: Gupta BS, Gupta U, eds. *Caffeine and Behavior: Current Views and Research Trends*. Boca Raton, FL: CRC Press. Pp. 1–16.

de Angelis L, Bertolissi M, Nardini G, Traversa U, Vertua R. 1982. Interaction of caffeine with benzodiazepines: Behavioral effects in mice. *Arch Int Pharmacodyn Ther* 225:89–102.

Dews PB, O'Brien CP, Bergman J. In press. Behavioral effects of caffeine: Dependence and related issues. In: *Caffeine and Health*. Washington, DC: ILSI North America.

Dimpfel W, Schober F, Spuler M. 1993. The influence of caffeine on human EEG under resting conditions and during mental loads. *Clin Investig* 71:197–207.

Dinges DF. 1989. Napping patterns and effects on human adults. In: Dinges DF, Broughton RJ, eds. *Sleep and Alertness: Chronobiological, Behavioral and Medical Aspects of Napping*. New York: Raven Press. Pp. 171–204.

Dinges DF, Orne MT, Whitehouse WG, Orne EC. 1987. Temporal placement of naps for alertness: Contributions of circadian phase and prior wakefulness. *Sleep* 10:313–329.

Dlugosz L, Bracken MB. 1992. Reproductive effects of caffeine: A review and theoretical analysis. *Epidemiol Rev* 14:83–100.

Dodd SL, Brooks E, Powers SK, Tulley R. 1991. The effects of caffeine on graded exercise performance in caffeine naive versus habituated subjects. *Eur J Appl Physiol* 62:424–429.

Dodd SL, Herb RA, Powers SK. 1993. Caffeine and exercise performance. An update. *Sports Med* 15:14–23.

Dreisbach RH. 1974. *Handbook of Poisoning: Diagnosis and Treatment*, 8th ed. Los Altos, CA: Lange Medical Publications.

Duke JA. 1988. *Handbook of Medicinal Herbs*. Boca Raton, FL: CRC Handbook Press. Pp. 131–132.

Durlach PJ. 1998. The effect of low dose caffeine on cognitive performance. *Psychopharmacology* 140:116–119.

Edgar DM, Seidel WF. 1997. Modafinil induces wakefulness without intensifying motor activity or subsequent rebound hypersomnolence in the rat. *J Pharmacol Exp Ther* 283:757–769.

Eggertsen R, Andreasson A, Hedner T, Karlberg BE, Hansson L. 1993. Effect of coffee on ambulatory blood pressure in patients with hypertension. *J Intern Med* 233:351–355.

Emonson DL, Vanderbeek RD. 1995. The use of amphetamines in U.S. Air Force tactical operations during Desert Shield and Storm. *Aviat Space Environ Med* 66:260–263.

Erickson MA, Schwarzkoff RJ, McKenzie RD. 1987. Effects of caffeine, fructose, and glucose ingestion on muscle glycogen utilization during exercise. *Med Sci Sports Exerc* 19:579–583.

Eskenazi B, Stapleton AL, Kharrazi M, Chee WY. 1999. Associations between maternal decaffeinated and caffeinated coffee consumption and fetal growth and gestational duration. *Epidemiology* 10:242–249.

Essig, D, Costill DL, Van Handel PJ. 1980. Effects of caffeine ingestion on utilization of muscle glycogen and lipid during leg ergometer cycling. *Int J Sports Med* 1:86–90.

Falk JL, Lau CE. 1991. Synergism of caffeine and by cocaine of the motor control deficit produced by midazolam. In: Gupta BS, Gupta U, eds. *Caffeine and Behavior: Current Views and Research Trends*. Boca Raton, FL: CRC Press. P. 78.

Falk B, Burstein R, Rosenblum J, Shapiro Y, Zylber-Katz E, Bashan N. 1990. Effects of caffeine ingestion on body fluid balance and thermoregulation during exercise. *Can J Physiol Pharmacol* 68:889–892.

FDA (Food and Drug Administration). 1980a. *Caffeine Content of Various Products*. Talk Paper T80-45, October 9. Rockville, MD: FDA.

FDA. 1980b. Proposed rule making. Removal of caffeine from GRAS list. *Federal Register* 45:69817.

FDA. 1987. Caffeine in nonalcoholic carbonated beverages. *Federal Register* 52:18923–18926.

FDA. 1999. Schedules of controlled substances: Placement of modafinil into schedule IV. Final rule. *Federal Register* 64:4050–4052.

Fenster L, Quale C, Waller K, Windham GC, Elkin EP, Benowitz N, Swan SH. 1999. Caffeine consumption and menstrual function. *Am J Epidemiol* 149:550–557.

Fernandes O, Sabharwal M, Smiley T, Pastuszak A, Koren G, Einarson T. 1998. Moderate to heavy caffeine consumption during pregnancy and relationship to spontaneous abortion and abnormal fetal growth: A meta-analysis. *Reprod Toxicol* 12:435–444.

Finn IB, Holtzman SG. 1986. Tolerance to caffeine-induced stimulation of locomotor activity in rats. *J Pharmacol Exp Ther* 238:542–545.

Flinn S, Gregory J, McNaughton LR, Tristram S, Davies P. 1990. Caffeine ingestion prior to incremental cycling to exhaustion in recreational cyclists. *Int J Sports Med* 11:188–193.

Foreman N, Barraclough S, Moore C, Mehta A, Madon M. 1989. High doses of caffeine impair performance of a numerical version of the Stroop Task in men. *Pharmocol Biochem Behav* 32:399–403.

Fulco CS, Rock PB, Trad LA, Rose MS, Forte VA Jr, Young PM, Cymerman A. 1994. Effect of caffeine on submaximal exercise performance at altitude. *Aviat Space Environ Med* 65:539–545.

Gander PH, Gregory KB, Miller DL, Graeber RC, Connell LJ, Rosekind MR. 1998. Flight crew fatigue V: Long-haul air transport operation. *Aviat Space Environ Med* 69:B37–B48.

Gastin PB, Miesner JE, Boileau RA, Slaughter MH. 1990. Failure of caffeine to enhance exercise performance in incremental treadmill running. *Aust J Sci Med Sports* 22:23–27.

George J, Murphy T, Roberts R, Cooksley WGE, Halliday KW, Powell LW. 1986. Influence of alcohol and caffeine consumption on caffeine elimination. *Clin Exp Pharmacol Physiol* 13:731–736.

Ghai G, Zimmerman MB, Hopkins MF. 1987. Evidence for A1 and A2 adenosine receptors in guinea pig trachea. *Life Sci* 41:1215–1224.

Gilman AG, Rall TW, Nies AS, Taylor P (eds). 1990. In: *Goodman and Gilman's The Pharmacological Bases of Therapeutics in Two Volumes*. New York: McGraw-Hill. P. 625.

Glynn NW, Meilahn EN, Charron M, Anderson SJ, Kuller LH, Cauley JA. 1995. Determinants of bone mineral density in older men. *J Bone Miner Res* 10:1769–1777.

Gold LH, Balster RL. 1996. Evaluation of the cocaine-like discriminative stimulus effects and reinforcing effects of modafinil. *Psychopharmacology* 126:286–292.

Goldstein A, Warren R, Kaizer S. 1965. Psychotropic effects of caffeine in man. I. Individual differences in sensitivity to caffeine-induced wakefulness. *J Pharmacol Exp Ther* 149:156–159.

Gomez S, Kelly T, Schlangen K, Elsmore T, Engelland RS. 1993. Improvement in cognitive performance after the administration of a single dose of pemoline during a 64-hr period without sleep. *J Sleep Res* 22:331.

Gonzalez-Alonso J, Heaps CL, Coyle EF. 1992. Rehydration after exercise with common beverages and water. *Int J Sports Med* 13:399–406.

Gordon NF, Myburgh JL, Kruger PE, Kempff PG, Cilliers JF, Moolman J, Grobler HC. 1982. Effects of caffeine ingestion on thermoregulatory and myocardial function during endurance performance. *S Afr Med J* 62:644–647.

Graham TE, Spriet LL. 1995. Metabolic, catecholamine, and exercise performance response to various doses of caffeine. *J Appl Physiol* 78:867–874.

Graham TE, Rush JWE, van Soeren MH. 1994. Caffeine and exercise: Metabolism and performance. *Can J Appl Physiol* 19:111–138.

Grand AN, Bell LN. 1997. Caffeine content of fountain and private-label store brand carbonated beverages. *J Am Diet Assoc* 97:179–182.

Grant DM, Campbell ME, Tang BK, Kalow W. 1987. Biotransformation of caffeine by microsomes from human liver. Kinetics and inhibition studies. *Biochem Pharmacol* 36:1251–1260.

Green HJ, Symon S, Daley R. 1990. Attenuation of human quadriceps fatigue with caffeine. *Can J Appl Sports Sci* 15:115.

Green PJ, Suls J. 1996. The effects of caffeine on ambulatory blood pressure, heart rate, and mood in coffee drinkers. *J Behav Med* 19:111–128.

Greenberg W, Shapiro D. 1987. The effects of caffeine and stress on blood pressure in individuals with and without a family history of hypertension. *Psychophysiology* 24:151–156.

Griffiths RR, Mumford KG. 1995. Caffeine—A drug of abuse? In: Bloom EF, Kupfer JD, eds. *Psychopharmacology: The Fourth Generation of Progress*. New York: Raven Press. Pp. 1699–1713.

Griffiths RR, Woodson PP. 1988. Caffeine physical dependence: A review of human and laboratory animal studies. *Psychopharmacology* 94:437–451.

Griffiths RR, Bigelow GE, Liebson IA. 1986. Human coffee drinking: Reinforcing and physical dependence producing effects of caffeine. *J Pharmacol Exp Ther* 239:416–425.

Griffiths RR, Evans SM, Heishman SJ, Preston KL, Sannerud CA, Wolf B, Woodson PP. 1990. Low-dose caffeine physical dependence in humans. *J Pharmacol Exp Ther* 255:1123–1132.

Haller CA, Benowitz NL. 2000. Adverse cardiovascular and central nervous system events associated with dietary supplements containing ephedra alkaloids. *N Engl J Med* 343:1833–1838.

Heaney RP. In press. Effects of caffeine on bone and the calcium economy. In: *Caffeine and Health*. Washington, DC: ILSI North America.

Heaney RP, Recker RR. 1982. Effects of nitrogen, phosphorus, and caffeine on calcium balance in women. *J Lab Clin Med* 99:46–55.

Heishman SJ, Henningfield JE. 1992. Stimulus functions of caffeine in humans: Relation to dependence potential. *Neurosci Biobehav Rev* 16:273–287.

Heishman SJ, Henningfield JE. 1994. Is caffeine a drug of dependence? Criteria and comparisons. *Pharmacopsychoecologia* 7:127–135.

Hermant J-F, Rambert FA, Duteil J. 1991. Awakening properties of modafinil: Effect on nocturnal activities in monkeys (*Macaca mulatta*) after acute and repeated administration. *Psychopharmacology* 103:28–32.

Hernandez-Avila M, Colditz GA, Stampfer MJ, Rosner B, Speizer FE, Willett WC. 1991. Caffeine, moderate alcohol intake, and risk of fractures of the hip and forearm in middle-aged women. *Am J Clin Nutr* 54:157–163.

Hetzler RK, Knowlton RG, Somani SM, Brown DD, Perkins RM III. 1990. Effect of parazantine on FFA mobilization after intravenous caffeine administration in humans. *J Appl Physiol* 68:44–47.

Hodgman MJ. 1998. Caffeine. In: Wexler P, ed. *Encyclopedia of Toxicology*. San Diego: Academic Press. Pp. 209–210.

Höfer I, Bättig K. 1993. Coffee consumption, blood pressure tonus and reactivity to physical challenge in 338 women. *Pharmacol Biochem Behav* 44:573–576.

Hogervorst E, Riedel WJ, Schmitt JA, Jolles J. 1998. Caffeine improves memory performance during distraction in middle-aged, but not in young or old subjects. *Human Psychopharmocol* 13:277–284.

Hogervorst E, Riedel WJ, Kovacs E, Brouns F, Jolles J. 1999. Caffeine improves cognitive performance after strenuous physical exercise. *Int J Sports Med* 20:354–361.

Holtzman SG, Mante S, Minneman KP. 1991. Role of adenosine receptors in caffeine tolerance. *J Pharmacol Exp Ther* 256:62–81.

Horne JA, Reyner LA. 1996. Counteracting driver sleepiness: Effect of napping, caffeine, and placebo. *Psychophysiology* 33:306–309.

Horton TJ, Geissler CA. 1996. Post-prandial thermogenesis with ephedrine, caffeine and aspirin in lean pre-disposed obese and obese women. *Int J Obes Relat Metab Disord* 20:91–97.

Iancu I, Dolberg OT, Zohar J. 1996. Is caffeine involved in the pathogenesis of combat-stress reaction? *Mil Med* 161:230–232.

IFT (Institute of Food Technologists). 1983. Expert Panel on Food Safety and Nutrition. Caffeine: A Scientific Status Summary. Chicago: IFT.

IOM (Institute of Medicine). 1993. Nutritional Needs in Hot Environments: Applications for Military Personnel in Field Operations. Washington, DC: National Academy Press.

IOM. 1994. *Food Components to Enhance Performance.* Washington, DC: National Academy Press.

IOM. 1996. Nutritional Needs in Cold and High-Altitude Environments. Washington, DC: National Academy Press.

IOM. 1999. Military Strategies for Sustainment of Nutrition and Immune Function in the Field. Washington, DC: National Academy Press.

Jackman M, Wendling P, Friars D, Graham TE. 1996. Metabolic catecholamine and endurance responses to caffeine during intense exercise. *J Appl Physiol* 81:1658–1663.

James JE. 1990. The influence of user status and anxious disposition on the hypertensive effects of caffeine. *Int J Psychophysiol* 10:171–179.

James JE. 1994. Does caffeine enhance or merely restore degraded psychomotor performance? *Neuropsychobiology* 30:124–125.

James JE. 1995. Caffeine and psychomotor performance revisited. *Neuropsychobiology* 31:202–203.

James JE. 1998. Acute and chronic effects of caffeine on performance, mood, headache, and sleep. *Neuropsychobiology* 38:32–41.

Jarvis MJ. 1993. Does caffeine intake enhance levels of cognitive performance? *Psychopharmacology* 110:45–52.

Jee SH, He J, Whelton PK, Suh I, Klag MJ. 1999. The effect of chronic coffee drinking on blood pressure: A meta-analysis of controlled clinical trials. *Hypertension* 33:647–652.

Jensen TK, Henriksen TB, Hjollund NH, Scheike T, Kolstad H, Giwercman A, Ernst E, Bonde JP, Skakkebaek NE, Olsen J. 1998. Caffeine intake and fecundability: A follow-up study among 430 Danish couples planning their first pregnancy. *Reprod Toxicol* 12:289–295.

Johnson R. 1999. *Caffeine and Sentry Duty Performance.* Presented at the Institute of Medicine Workshop on Caffeine Formulations for Sustainment of Mental Task Performance During Military Operations, Washington, DC, February 2–3. Committee on Military Nutrition Research.

Kamimori GH, Joubert A, Otterstetter R, Santaromana M, Eddington ND. 1999. The effect of the menstrual cycle on the pharmacokinetics of caffeine in normal, healthy eumenorrheic females. *Eur J Clin Pharmacol* 55:445–449.

Kaplan GB, Greenblatt DJ, Ehrenberg BL, Goddard JE, Cotreau MM, Harmatz JS, Shader RI. 1997. Dose-dependent pharmacokinetics and psychomotor effects of caffeine in humans. *J Clin Pharmacol* 37:693–703.

Kautz MA. 1999. *Cognitive Performance Effects of Caffeine Versus Amphetamine Following Sleep Deprivation.* Presented at the Institute of Medicine Workshop on Caffeine Formulations for Sustainment of Mental Task Performance During Military Operations, Washington, DC, February 2–3. Committee on Military Nutrition Research.

Kawachi I, Colditz GA, Stone CB. 1994. Does coffee drinking increase the risk of coronary heart disease? Results from a meta-analysis. *Br Heart J* 72:269–275.

Kelly TL, Gomez S, Ryman D, McGeoy S, Rubin RT, Bonnet MH, Naitoh P. 1996. *Effects of Repeated Doses of Caffeine During 64 Hours of Sleep Deprivation on Subsequent Recovery Sleep.* Technical Report No. 96–11. San Diego: Naval Health Research Center.

Kenemans JL, Lorist MM. 1995. Caffeine and selective visual processing. *Pharmacol Biochem Behav* 52:461–471.

Kerr JS, Sherwood N, Hindmarch I. 1991. Separate and combined effects of the social drugs on psychomotor performance. In: Gupta BS, Gupta U, eds. *Caffeine and Behavior: Current Views and Research Trends.* Boca Raton, FL: CRC Press. P. 77.

Kiel DP, Felson DT, Hannan MT, Anderson JJ, Wilson WFP. 1990. Caffeine and the risk of hip fracture: The Framingham Study. *Am J Epidemiol* 132:675–683.

Kiyohara C, Kono S, Honjo S, Todoroki I, Sakurai Y, Nishiwaki M, Hamada H, Nishikawa H, Koga H, Ogawa S, Nakagawa K. 1999. Inverse association between coffee drinking and serum uric acid concentrations in middle-aged Japanese males. *Br J Nutr* 82:125–130.

Klebanoff MA, Levine RJ, DerSimonian R, Clemens JD, Wilkins DG. 1999. Maternal serum paraxanthine, a caffeine metabolite, and the risk of spontaneous abortion. *N Engl J Med* 341:1639–1644.

Kovacs EMR, Stegen JHCH, Brouns F. 1998. Effect of caffeinated drinks on substrate metabolism, caffeine excretion, and performance. *J Appl Physiol* 85:709–715.

Kuribara H, Tadokoro S. 1992. Caffeine does not effectively ameliorate, but rather may worsen the ethanol intoxication when assessed by discrete avoidance in mice. In: Gupta BS, Gupta U, eds. *Caffeine and Behavior: Current Views and Research Trends.* Boca Raton, FL: CRC Press. P. 50.

Kuznicki JT, Turner LS. 1986. The effects of caffeine on caffeine users and non-users. *Physiol Behav* 37:397–408.

Kynast-Gales SA, Massey LK. 1994. Effect of caffeine on circadian excretion of urinary calcium and magnesium. *J Am Coll Nutr* 13:467–472.

Lader MH. 1999. Caffeine withdrawal. In: Gupta BS, Gupta U, eds. *Caffeine and Behavior.* Boca Raton, FL: CRC Press. Pp. 151–159.

Lancaster T, Muir J, Silagy C. 1994. The effects of coffee on serum lipids and blood pressure in a UK population. *J Roy Soc Med* 87:506–507.

Lane JD, Adcock RA, Williams RB, Kuhn CM. 1990. Caffeine effects on cardiovascular and neuroendocrine responses to acute psychosocial stress and their relationship to level of habitual caffeine consumption. *Psychosom Med* 52:320–336.

Lane JD, Phillips-Bute BG, Pieper CF. 1998. Caffeine raises blood pressure at work. *Psychosom Med* 60:327–330.

Langer DH, Sweeney KP, Bartenbach DP, Davis PM, Menander KB. 1986. Evidence of lack of abuse or dependence following pemoline treatment: Results of a retrospective survey. *Drug Alcohol Depend* 17:213–227.

Laurent D, Schneider KE, Prusaczyk WK, Franklin C, Vogel SM, Krssak M, Petersen KF, Goforth HW, Shulman GI. 2000. Effects of caffeine on muscle glycogen utilization and the neuroendocrine axis during exercise. *J Clin Endocrin Metab* 85:2170–2175.

Lee EHY, Tsai MJ, Tang YP, Chai CY. 1987. Differential biochemical mechanisms mediate locomotor stimulation effects by caffeine and nicotine in rats. *Pharmacol Biochem Behav* 26:427–430.

Leviton A. 1993. *Reproductive Hazards in Humans.* In: Garattini S, ed. *Caffeine, Coffee, and Health.* New York: Raven Press. Pp. 343–358.

Leviton A. 1998. Caffeine consumption and the risk of reproductive hazards. *J Reprod Med* 33:175–178.

Lewis CE, Caan B, Funkhouser E, Hilner JE, Bragg C, Dyer A, Raczynski JM, Savage PJ, Armstrong MA, Friedman GD. 1993. Inconsistent associations of caffeine-containing beverages with blood pressure and lipoproteins. *Am J Epidemiol* 138:502–507.

Lieberman HR. 1992. Caffeine. In: Jones D, Smith A, eds. *Factors Affecting Human Performance*, Vol. II. London: Academic Press. Pp. 49–72.

Lieberman H. 1999. *Effect of Caffeine on Cognitive Function and Alertness*. Presented at the Institute of Medicine Workshop on Caffeine Formulations for Sustainment of Mental Task Performance During Military Operations, Washington, DC, February 2–3. Committee on Military Nutrition Research.

Lieberman HR, Wurtman RJ, Emde GG, Roberts C, Coviella ILG. 1987. The effects of low doses of caffeine on human performance and mood. *Psychopharmacology* 92:308–312.

Liguori A, Huges JR, Grass JA. 1997. Absorption and subjective effects of caffeine from coffee, cola, and capsules. *Pharmacol Biochem Behav* 58:721–726.

Lin JS, Roussel B, Akaoka H, Fort P, Debilly G, Jouvet M. 1992. Role of catecholamines in the modafinil and amphetamine induced wakefulness, a comparative pharmacological study in the cat. *Brain Res* 591:319–326.

Lin JS, Hou Y, Jouvet M. 1996. Potential brain neuronal targets for amphetamine-, methylphenidate-, and modafinil-induced wakefulness, evidenced by *c-fos* immunocytochemistry in the cat. *Proc Natl Acad Sci* 93:14128–14133.

Linde L. 1995. Mental effects of caffeine in fatigued and non-fatigued female and male subjects. *Ergonomics* 38:864–885.

Lloyd T, Rollings N, Eggli DF, Kieselhorst K, Chinchilli VM. 1997. Dietary caffeine intake and bone status of postmenopausal women. *Am J Clin Nutr* 65:1826–1830.

Lloyd T, Rollings NJ, Kieselhorst K, Eggli DF, Mauger E. 1998. Dietary caffeine intake is not correlated with adolescent bone gain. *J Am Coll Nutr* 17:454–457.

Lopes JM, Aubier M, Jardim J, Arnada VJ, Macklem PT. 1983. Effect of caffeine on skeletal muscle function before and after fatigue. *J Appl Physiol* 54:1303–1305.

Lopez F, Miller LG, Greenblatt DJ, Kaplan GB, Shader RI. 1989. Interaction of caffeine with the $GABA_A$ receptor complex: Alterations in receptor function but not ligand binding. In: Gupta BS, Gupta U, eds. *Caffeine and Behavior: Current Views and Research Trends*. Boca Raton, FL: CRC Press. P. 80.

Lorist MM, Snel J. 1997. Caffeine effects on perceptual and motor processes. *Electroencephalogr Clin Neurophysiol* 102:401–413.

Lorist MM, Snel J, Kok A. 1994a. Influence of caffeine on information processing stages in well-rested and fatigued subjects. *Psychopharmacology* 113:411–421.

Lorist MM, Snel J, Kok A, Mulder G. 1994b. Influence of caffeine on selective attention in well-rested and fatigued subjects. *Psychophysiology* 31:525–534.

Lovallo RL, Sung BH, Everson SA, Passey RB, Wilson MF. 1991. Hypertension risk and caffeine's effect on cardiovascular activity during mental stress in young men. *Health Psychology* 10:236–243.

Lovallo WR, al'Absi M, Pincomb GA, Everson SA, Sung BH, Passey RB, Wilson MF. 1996. Caffeine and behavioral stress effects on blood pressure in borderline hypertensive Caucasian men. *Health Psychol* 15:11–17.

MacDonald TM, Sharpe K, Fowler G, Lyons D, Freestone S, Lovell HG, Webster J, Petrie JC. 1991. Caffeine restriction: Effect on blood pressure. *Br Med J* 303:1235–1238.

Massey LK, Hollingbery PW. 1988. Acute effects of dietary caffeine and aspirin on urinary mineral excretion in pre- and postmenopausal women. *Nutr Res* 8:845–851.

Massey LK, Wise KJ. 1984. The effect of dietary caffeine on urinary excretion of calcium, magnesium, sodium and potassium in healthy young females. *Nutr Res* 4:43–50.

Massey LK, Bergman EA, Wise KJ, Sherrard DJ. 1989. Dietary caffeine lowers serum ultrafilterable calcium and raises bone alkaline phosphatase in older women consuming low dietary calcium. *J Bone Miner Res* 4:245.

Mathew RJ, Wilson WH. 1985. Caffeine consumption, withdrawal and cerebral blood flow. *Headache* 25:305–309.

Mathew RJ, Barr DL, Weinman ML. 1983. Caffeine and cerebral blood flow. *Br J Psychiatry* 143:604–608.

Mattila ME, Matilla MJ, Nuotto E. 1992. Caffeine moderately antagonizes the effects of triazolam and zopiclone on the psychomotor performance of healthy subjects. *Pharmacol Toxicol* 70:286–289.

Mattila MJ, Palva E, Savolainen K. 1992. Caffeine antagonizes diazepam effects in man. *Med Biol* 60:121–123.

Maughan RJ, Leiper JB. 1994. Post-exercise rehydration in man: Effect of voluntary intake of four different beverages. *Med Sci Sports Exerc* 25:S2.

McClellan KL, Spencer CM. 1998. Modafinil: A review of its pharmacology and clinical efficacy in the management of narcolepsy. In: *CNS Drugs* (4). Auckland, NZ: Adis International Limited. Pp. 311–324.

McNaughton LR. 1986. The influence of caffeine ingestion on incremental treadmill running. *Br J Sports Med* 20:109–112.

McPherson PS, Kim YK, Valdivia H, Knudson CM, Takekura H, Fanzini-Armstrong C, Coronado R, Campbell KP. 1991. The brain ryanodine receptor: A caffeine-sensitive calcium release channel. *Neuron* 71:17–25.

Mitchell PJ, Redman JR. 1992. Effects of caffeine, time of day and user history on study-related performance. *Psychopharmacology* 109:121–126.

Moachon G, Kammacher I, Clenet M, Matinier D. 1996. Pharmacokinetic profile of modafinil. *Drugs Today* 32:327–337.

Molina J, Orsinger K. 1990. Dopaminergic effects of pemoline. *Brain Res* 80:52–57.

Murphy TL, McIvor G, Yap A, Cooksley WGE, Halliday JW, Powell LW. 1988. The effect of smoking on caffeine elimination: Implication for its use as a semiquantitative test of liver function. *Clin Exp Pharmacol Physiol* 15:9–13.

Myers HF, Shapiro D, McClure F, Daims R. 1989. Impact of caffeine and psychological stress on blood pressure in black and white men. *Health Psychol* 8:597–612.

Myers JP, Johnson DA, McVey DE. 1999. Caffeine and the modulation of brain function. In: Gupta BS, Gupta U, eds. *Caffeine and Behavior: Current Views and Research Trends.* Boca Raton, FL: CRC Press. Pp. 17–30.

Myers MG. In press. Cardiovascular effects of caffeine. In: *Caffeine and Health.* Washington, DC: ILSI North America.

Myers MG, Basinski A. 1992. Coffee and coronary heart disease. *Arch Intern Med* 152:1767–1772.

Naismith DJ, Akinyanju PA, Szanto S, Yudkin J. 1970. The effect in volunteers of coffee and decaffeinated coffee on blood glucose, insulin, plasma lipids, and some factors involved with blood clotting. *Nutr Metab* 12:144–151.

Naitoh P, Kelly TL, Babkoff H. 1992. Napping, stimulant, and four-choice performance. In: Broughton RJ, Oglivie RD, eds. *Sleep, Arousal, and Performance.* Boston: Birkhäuser.

Nehlig A, Daval JL, Pereira de Vasconcelos A, Boyet S. 1987. Caffeine-diazepam interaction and local cerebral glucose utilization in the conscious rat. *Brain Res* 419:272–278.

Nehlig A, Daval JL, Derby G. 1992. Caffeine and the central nervous system: Mechanisms and action, biochemical, and psychostimulant effects. *Brain Res Rev* 17:139–170.

Neuhauser-Berthold M, Beine S, Verwied SC, Luhrmann PM. 1997. Coffee consumption and total body water homeostasis as measured by fluid balance and bioelectrical impedance analysis. *Ann Nutr Metab* 41:29–36.

Newby EE, Neilson JM, Jarvie DR, Boon NA. 1996. Caffeine restricion has no role in the management of patients with symptomatic idiopathic ventricular premature beats. *Heart* 76:335–337.

Newhouse PA, Belenky G, Thomas M, Thorne D, Sing HC, Fertig J. 1989. The effects of d-amphetamine on arousal, cognition, and mood after prolonged total sleep deprivation. *Neuropsychopharmacology* 2:153–164.

Nicholson AN, Pascoe PA. 1989. Dopaminergic transmission and the sleep-wakefulness continuum in man. *Neuropharmacology* 29:411–417.

Nicholson AN, Turner C. 1998. Intensive and sustained air operations: Potential use of the stimulant, pemoline. *J Aviat Space Environ Med* 69:647–655.

Nicholson AN, Stone BM, Jones MM. 1980. Wakefulness and reduced rapid eye movement sleep: Studies with prolintane and pemoline. *Br J Clin Pharmacol* 10:465–472.

Nicolaidis S, De Saint Hilaire Z. 1993. Nonamphetamine awakening agent modafinil induces feeding changes in the rat. *Brain Res Bull* 32:87–90.

Nurminen ML, Niitynen L, Korpela R, Vapaatalo H. 1999. Coffee, caffeine and blood pressure: A critical review. *Eur J Clin Nutr* 53:831–839.

Nussberger J, Mooser V, Maridor G, Juillerat L, Waeber B. Brunner HR. 1990. Caffeine-induced diuresis and atrial natriuretic peptides. *J Cardiovasc Phamacol* 15:635–691.

Packard PT, Recker RR. 1996. Caffeine does not affect the rate of gain in spine bone in young women. *Osteoporosis Int* 6:149–152.

Parsons WD, Neims AH. 1978. Effect of smoking on caffeine clearance. *Clin Pharmacol Ther* 24:40–45.

Pasman WJ, van Baak MA, Jeukendrup AE, de Haan A. 1995. The effect of different dosages of caffeine on endurance performance time. *Int J Sports Med* 16:225–230.

Patwardhan RV, Desmond PV, Johnson RF, Schenker S. 1980. Impaired elimination of caffeine by oral contraceptive steroid. *J Lab Clin Med* 95:603–608.

Penetar D. 1999. *General Overview of Military Interest and Research on Role of Caffeine in Physical and Cognitive Performance*. Presented at the Institute of Medicine Workshop on Caffeine Formulations for Sustainment of Mental Task Performance During Military Operations, Washington, DC, February 2–3. Committee on Military Nutrition Research.

Penetar DM, McCann U, Thorne D, Kamimori G, Galinski C, Sing H, Thomas M, Belenky G. 1993. Caffeine reversal of sleep deprivation effects on alertness and mood. *Psychopharmacology* 112:359–365.

Penetar DM, McCann U, Thorne D, Schelling A, Galinski C, Sing H, Thomas M, Belenky G. 1994. Effects of caffeine on cognitive performance, mood and alertness in sleep-deprived humans. In: Institute of Medicine. *Food Components to Enhance Performance*. Washington, DC: National Academy Press. Pp. 407–431.

Perod AL, Roberts AE, McKinney WM. 2000. Caffeine can affect velocity in the middle cerebral artery during hyperventilation, hypoventilation, and thinking: A transcranial doppler study. *J Neuroimaging* 10:33–38.

Persson CA, Karlsson JA, Erjefalt I. 1982. Differentiation among bronchodilation and universal adenosine antagonism among xanthine derivatives. *Life Sci* 30:2181–2189.

Piérard C, Satabin P, Lagarde D, Barrère B, Guezennec CY, Menu JP, Pérès M. 1995. Effects of vigilance-enhancing drug, modafinil, on rat brain metabolism: A 2D COSY ^{1}H-NMR study. *Brain Res* 693:251–256.

Pigeau R, Naitoh P, Buguet A, McCann C, Baranski J, Taylor M, Thompson M, Mack I. 1995. Modafinil, d-amphetamine and placebo during 64 hours of sustained mental work. I. Effects on mood, fatigue, cognitive performance and body temperature. *J Sleep Res* 4:212–228.

Pincomb GA, Lovallo WR, Passey RB, Brackett DJ, Wilson MF. 1987. Caffeine enhances the physiological response to occupational stress in medical students. *Health Psychol* 6:101–102.

Pirich C, O'Grady J, Sinzinger H. 1993. Coffee, lipoproteins and cardiovascular disease. *Wien Klin Wochenschr* 105:3–6.

Pollard I, Murray JF, Hiller R, Scaramuzzi RJ, Wilson CA. 1999. Effects of preconceptual caffeine. *J Matern Fetal Med* 8:220–224.

Pollock BG, Wylie M, Stack JA, Sorisio DA, Thompson DS, Kirshner MA, Folan MM, Condifer KA. 1999. Inhibition of caffeine metabolism by estrogen replacement therapy in postmenopausal women. *J Clin Pharmacol* 39:936–940.

Polson JB, Krzanowski JJ, Szentvanyi A. 1985. Correlation between inhibition of a cyclic GMP phosphodiesterase and relaxation of canine tracheal smooth muscle. *Biochem Pharmacol* 34:1875–1879.

Porkka-Heiskanen T. 1999. Adenosine in sleep and wakefulness. *Ann Med* 31:125–129.

Porkka-Heiskanen T, Streeker RE, Thakkar M, Bjorkum AA, Greene RW, McCarley RW. 1997. Adenosine: A mediator of the sleep-inducing effects of prolonged wakefulness. *Science* 276:1235–1268.

Prusaczyk WK. 1999. *Caffeine Research in the Navy*. Presented at the Institute of Medicine Workshop on Caffeine Formulations for Sustainment of Mental Task Performance During Military Operations, Washington, DC, February 2–3. Committee on Military Nutrition Research.

Purves D, Sullivan FM. 1993. Reproductive effects of caffeine. In: Cerattini S, ed. *Caffeine, Coffee, and Health*. New York: Raven Press, Ltd. P. 317.

Rees K, Allen D, Lader M. 1999. The influences of age and caffeine on psychomotor and cognitive function. *Psychopharmacology (Berl)* 14592:191–188.

Reeves RR, Strune FA, Patrick G, Bullen JA. 1995. Topographic quantitative EEG measures of alpha and theta power changes during caffeine withdrawal: Preliminary findings from normal subjects. *Clin Encephalogr* 26:154–162.

Reyner LA, Horne JA. 2000. Early morning driver sleepiness: Effectiveness of 200 mg caffeine. *Psychophysiology* 37:251–256.

Robertson D, Wade D, Workman R, Woosley RL, Oates JA. 1981. Tolerance to humoral and hemodynamic effects of caffeine in man. *J Clin Invest* 67:1111–1117.

Rogers PJ, Dernoncourt C. 1998. Regular caffeine consumption: A balance of adverse and beneficial effects for mood and psychomotor performance. *Pharmacol Biochem Behav* 59:1039–1045.

Rogers PJ, Richardson NJ, Dernoncourt C. 1995. Caffeine use: Is there a net benefit for mood and psychomotor performance? *Neuropsychobiology* 31:195–199.

Rosenthal L, Roehrs T, Zwyghuizen-Doorenbos A, Plath D, Roth T. 1991. Alerting effects of caffeine after normal and restricted sleep. *Neuropsychopharmacology* 4:103–108.

Rossignol AM. 1985. Caffeine-containing beverages and premenstrual syndrome in young women. *Am J Public Health* 75:1335–1337.

Sallee FR, Stiller RL, Perel JM. 1992. Pharmacodynamics of pemoline in attention deficit disorder with hyperactivity. *J Am Acad Child Adolesc Psychiatry* 31:244–251.

Sansone M, Battaglia M, Castellano C. 1994. Effect of caffeine and nicotine on avoidance learning in mice: Lack of interaction. *J Pharm Pharmacol* 46:765–767.

Santos IS, Victora CG, Huttly S, Carvalhal JB. 1998. Caffeine intake and low birth weight: A population-based case-control study. *Am J Epidemiol* 147:620–627.

Sasaki H, Maeda J, Usui S, Ishiko T. 1987. Effect of sucrose and caffeine ingestion on performance of prolonged strenuous running. *Int J Sports Med* 8:261–265.

Schmitz W, von der Leyen H, Meyer W, Neumann J, Scholtz H. 1989. Phosphodiesterase inhibition and positive ionotrophic effects. *J Cardiovasc Pharmacol* 14:511–514.

Sedor FA, Schneider KA, Heyden S. 1991. Effect of coffee on cholesterol and apolipoproteins, corroborated by caffeine levels. *Am J Prev Med* 7:391–396.

Senechal PK. 1988. Flight surgeon of combat operations at RAF Upper Heyford. *Aviat Space Environ Med* 59:776–777.

Sicard BA, Perault MC, Enslen M, Chauffard F, Vandel B, Tachon P. 1996. The effects of 600 mg of slow release caffeine on mood and alertness. *Aviat Space Environ Med* 67:859–862.

Silverman K, Evans SM, Strain EC, Griffiths RR. 1992. Withdrawal syndrome after the double-blind cessation of caffeine consumption. *N Engl J Med* 327:1109–1114.

Smith A, Rubin GH. 1999. *Positive Effects of Caffeine or Negative Effects of Caffeine Withdrawal*. Presented at the Institute of Medicine Workshop on Caffeine Formulations for Sustainment of Mental Task Performance During Military Operations, Washington, DC, February 2–3. Committee on Military Nutrition Research.

Smith S. 1999. *Caffeine to Counteract Performance Deficits Due to Sleep Deprivation*. Presented at the Institute of Medicine Workshop on Caffeine Formulations for Sustainment of Mental Task Performance During Military Operations, Washington, DC, February 2–3. Committee on Military Nutrition Research.

Spiegel R. 1979. Effects of amphetamines on performance, and on polygraphic sleep parameters in man. *Adv Biosci* 21:189–201.

Spielman WS, Arend LJ. 1991. Adenosine receptors and signaling in the kidney. *Hypertension* 17:117–130.

Spriet LL. 1995. Caffeine and performance. *Int J Sport Nutr* 5:S84–S99.

Spriet LL. 1999. *Caffeine and Muscle Metabolism During Prolonged Exercise*. Presented at the Institute of Medicine Workshop on Caffeine Formulations for Sustainment of Mental Task Performance During Military Operations, Washington, DC, February 2–3. Committee on Military Nutrition Research.

Spriet LL, MacLean DA, Dyck DJ, Hultman E, Cederblad G, Graham TE. 1992. Caffeine ingestion and muscle metabolism during prolonged exercise in humans. *Am J Physiol* 262:E891–E898.

Stamler J, Caggiula AW, Grandits GA. 1997. Relation of body mass and alcohol, nutrient, fiber, and caffeine intakes to blood pressure in the special intervention and usual care groups in the Multiple Risk Intervention Trial. *Am J Clin Nutr* 65:338S–365S.

Stamph C. 1989. Ultrashort sleep/wake patterns and sustained performance. In: Dinges DF, Broughton RI, eds. *Sleep and Alertness: Chronobiological, Behavioral and Medical Aspects of Napping*. New York: Raven Press. Pp. 139–170.

Stanton CK, Gray RH. 1995. Effects of caffeine consumption on delayed conception. *Am J Epidemiol* 142:1322–1329.

Stavric B. 1988. Methylaxanthines: Toxicity to humans, 3. Theobromine, paraxanthine and the combined effects of methylxanthines. *Food Chem Toxicol* 26:725–733.

Stivalet P, Esquivie D, Barraud P-A, Leifflen D, Raphel C. 1998. Effects of modafinil on attentional processes during 60 hours of sleep deprivation. *Hum Psychopharmacol Clin Exp* 13:501–507.

Streufert S, Satish U, Pogash R, Gingrich D, Landis R, Roache J, Severs W. 1997. Excess coffee consumption in simulated complex work settings: Detriment or facilitation of performance. *J Appl Psych* 82:774–782.

Stickgold R. 1999. *Eyelid Movement as a Physiological Predictor of Cognitive Impairment with Sleep Deprivation.* Presented at the Institute of Medicine Workshop on Caffeine Formulations for Sustainment of Mental Task Performance During Military Operations, Washington, DC, February 2–3. Committee on Military Nutrition Research.

Sung BH, Lovallo WR, Whitsett T, Wilson MF. 1995. Caffeine elevates blood pressure response to exercise in mild hypertensive men. *Am J Hyperten* 8:1184–1188.

Tarnopolsky MA. 1994. Caffeine and endurance performance. *Sports Med* 18:109–125.

Tarnopolsky MA, Atkinson SA, MacDougall JD, Sale DG, Sutton JR. 1989. Physiological responses to caffeine during endurance running in habitual caffeine users. *Med Sci Sports Exerc* 21:418–424.

Tarnopolsky MA, Hicks A, Cupido C, McComas AJ. 1992. Caffeine and neuromuscular function in humans: No effects of tolerance. *Physiologist* 35:201.

Tavani A, Negri E, La Vecchia C. 1995. Coffee intake and risk of hip fracture in women in northern Italy. *Prev Med* 24:396–400.

Urgert R, Katan MB. 1997. The cholesterol-raising factor from coffee beans. *Annu Rev Nutr* 17:305–324.

U.S. Air Force. 2001. *Policy Letter on Implementation, Combat Air Force Aircrew Fatigue Countermeasures.* Commander, Air Force Medical Operations, Office of the Surgeon General, Memorandum. June 26. Bolling Air Force Base, Washington, DC.

U.S. Navy. 2000. *Performance Maintenance During Continuous Flight Operations. A Guide for Flight Surgeons.* Performance Maintenance Manual, Naval Strike and Air Warfare Center. Pensacola, FL: Naval Operational Medicine Institute.

van Soeren MH, Sathasivam P, Spriet LL, Graham TE. 1993. Caffeine metabolism and epinephrine responses during exercise in users and nonusers. *J Appl Physiol* 75:805–812.

Vermeulen NP, Teunissen MWE, Breimer DD. 1979. Pharmacokinetics of pemoline in plasma, saliva and urine following oral administration. *Br J Clin Pharmacol* 8:459–463.

Walsh JK, Meuhlbach MJ, Humm TM, Dickens QS, Sugarman JL, Schweitzer PK. 1990. Effect of caffeine on physiological sleep tendency and ability to sustain wakefulness at night. *Psychopharmacology* 101:271–273.

Walsh JK, Meuhlbach MJ, Schweitzer PK. 1995. Hypnotics and caffeine as countermeasures for shift work-related sleepiness and sleep disturbance. *J Sleep Res* 4:S80–S83.

Waluga M, Janusz M, Karpel E, Hartleb M, Nowak A. 1998. Cardiovascular effects of ephedrine, caffeine and yohimbine measured by thoracic electrical bioimpedance in obese women. *Clin Physiol* 18:69–67.

Warburton DM. 1995. Effects of caffeine on cognition and mood without caffeine abstinence. *Psychopharmacology* 119:66–70.

Weber JG, Ereth MH, Danielson DR. 1993. Perioperative ingestion of caffeine and postoperative headache. *Mayo Clin Proc* 68:842–845.

Wei M, Macera CA, Hornung CA, Blair SN. 1995. The impact of changes in coffee consumption on serum cholesterol. *J Clin Epidemiol* 48:1189–1196.

Weir RL, Hruska RE. 1983. Interaction between methylzanthines and the benzodiazepine receptor. In: Gupta BS, Gupta U, eds. *Caffeine and Behavior: Current Views and Research Trends*. Boca Raton, FL: CRC Press. P. 19.

Wemple RD, Lamb DR, McKeever KH. 1997. Caffeine vs caffeine-free sports drinks: Effects on urine production at rest and during prolonged exercise. *Int J Sports Med* 18:40–46.

White JM. 1988. Behavioral interactions between nicotine and caffeine. *Pharmacol Behav* 29:63–66.

White JM. 1999. Behavioral effects of caffeine coadministered with nicotine, benzodiazepines, and alcohol. In: Gupta BS, Gupta U, eds. *Caffeine and Behavior*. Boca Raton, FL: CRC Press. Pp. 75–86.

Wiles JD, Bird SR, Hopkins J, Riley M. 1992. Effect of caffeinated coffee on running speed, respiratory factors, blood lactate and perceived exertion during 1500 m treadmill running. *Br J Sport Med* 26:116–120.

Willett WC, Stampfer MJ, Manson JE, Colditz GA, Rosner BA, Speizer FE, Hennekens CH. 1996. Coffee consumption and cornonary hart disease in women. A ten-year follow-up. *J Am Med Assoc* 275:458–462.

Williams RD. 1999. Healthy pregnancy, healthy baby. Exercise, good food, and prenatal care are the keys. *FDA Consumer* 33:18–22.

Wise KJ, Bergmon EA, Sherrad DJ, Massey LK. 1996. Interactions between dietary calcium and caffeine consumption on calcium metabolism in hypertensive humans. *Am J Hypertens* 9:223–229.

Wolfrom D, Welsh CW. 1990. Caffeine and the development of normal, benign and carcinomatous human breast tissues: A relationship? *J Med* 21:225–250.

Woodward M, Tunstall-Pedoe H. 1999. Coffee and tea consumption in the Scottish Heart Health Study follow-up: Conflicting relations with coronary risk factors, coronary disease, and all cause mortality. *J Epidemiol Community Health* 53:481–487.

Wyatt J. 1999. *Circadian and Sleep Homeostatic Modulation of Sleep and Performance*. Presented at the Institute of Medicine Workshop on Caffeine Formulations for Sustainment of Mental Task Performance During Military Operations, Washington, DC, February 2–3. Committee on Military Nutrition Research.

Youngstedt SD, O'Connor PJ, Crabbe JB, Dishman RK. 1998. Acute exercise reduces caffeine-induced anxiogenesis. *Med Sci Sports Exerc* 30:740–745.

Zahn TP, Rapoport J. 1987. Autonomic nervous system effects of acute doses of caffeine in caffeine users and abstainers. *Int J Psychophysiol* 5:33–41.

Zwyghuizen-Doorenbos A, Roehrs TA, Lipschietz L, Timms V, Roth T. 1990. Effects of caffeine on alertness. *Psychopharmacology* 100:36–39.

Appendixes

A

Workshop Agenda and Abstracts

AGENDA

Caffeine Formulations for Sustainment of Mental Task Performance During Military Operations

Committee on Military Nutrition Research
February 2–3, 1999

Tuesday February 2, 1999

8:30 a.m. Welcome on Behalf of the Food and Nutrition Board
Dr. Allison A. Yates, Director, Food and Nutrition Board

8:40 Welcome on Behalf of the Committee on Military Nutrition
Dr. John Vanderveen, Chair, Committee on Military Nutrition Research

8:45 Opening Comments on Behalf of the Military
LTC Karl E. Friedl, U.S. Army Medical Research and Materiel Command, Fort Detrick, Frederick, MD

Part I. Effects on Mental and Physical Performance
Moderator: Dr. Robin Kanarek

9:00 General Overview of Military Interest and Research on Role of Caffeine in Physical and Cognitive Performance
COL David Penetar, U.S. Army Research Institute of Environmental Medicine, Natick, MA

9:35 Caffeine and Muscle Metabolism During Prolonged Exercise
Dr. Lawrence Spriet, University of Guelph, Ontario, Canada

10:10	Effect of Caffeine on Cognitive Function and Alertness *Dr. Harris Lieberman, U.S. Army Research Institute of Environmental Medicine, Natick, MA*
10:45	BREAK
10:55	Caffeine and Sentry Duty Performance *Dr. Richard Johnson, U.S. Army Research Institute of Environmental Medicine, Natick, MA*
11:30	Eyelid Movement as a Physiological Predictor of Cognitive Impairment During Sleep Deprivation *Dr. Robert Stickgold, Harvard Medical School, Boston, MA*
12:05 p.m.	Circadian and Sleep Homeostatic Modulation of Sleep and Performance *Dr. James Wyatt, Harvard Medical School and Brigham and Women's Hospital, Boston, MA*
12:40	LUNCH

Moderator: Dr. Johanna Dwyer

1:45	Caffeine Effects During Sleep Deprivation and Recovery *Dr. Steven Smith, Pennington Biomedical Research Center, Louisiana State University, Baton Rouge, LA*
2:20	Circadian and Homeostatic Interactions in Waking Neurobehavioral Functions During Partial and Total Sleep Deprivation: Effects of Caffeine *Dr. Hans Van Dongen, University of Pennsylvania School of Medicine, Philadelphia*
2:55	Caffeine Research in the Navy *Dr. W.K. Prusaczyk, Naval Health Research Center, San Diego, CA*
3:30	DISCUSSION
3:50	BREAK

APPENDIX A

Part II. Safety Issues of Caffeine Supplementation
Moderator: Dr. John Fernstrom

4:00   Caffeine as a Model Drug of Abuse
       Dr. Steve Holtzman, Emory University School of Medicine, Atlanta, GA

4:35   Caffeine Physical Dependence and the Consequences of Caffeine Abstinence
       Dr. Roland Griffiths, Johns Hopkins University School of Medicine, Baltimore, MD

5:10   Positive Effects of Caffeine or Negative Effects of Withdrawal
       Dr. Andrew Smith, University of Bristol, United Kingdom

5:30   DISCUSSION

6:00   ADJOURN

Wednesday, February 3, 1999

Part III. Caffeine Dose and Formulations
Moderator: Dr. Gail Butterfield

9:00 a.m.   Pharmacology of Caffeine
            Dr. Gary Kamimori, Walter Reed Army Institute of Research, Washington, DC

9:35   Caffeine Usage on Submarines
        Christine Schlichting, Naval Submarine Medical Research Laboratory, Groton, CT

10:10   Design of a Food Matrix for the Delivery of Performance-Enhancing Components
        Dr. Jack Briggs, Natick Soldier Center, Natick, MA

10:45   BREAK

10:55   Caffeine and Carbohydrate Supplements for Physical Performance
        Dr. John Ivy, University of Texas, Austin

11:30   DISCUSSION

12:00 noon LUNCH

Part IV. Alternatives to Caffeine for Mental and Physical Task Performance
Moderator: Dr. Esther Sternberg

1:15 p.m. Cognitive Performance Effects of Caffeine Versus Amphetamines Following Sleep Deprivation
CAPT Mary Kautz, Walter Reed Army Institute of Research, Silver Spring, MD

1:50 Use of Amphetamine to Counteract Sleep Deprivation in Aviators
Dr. John Caldwell, U.S. Army Aeromedical Research Laboratory, Fort Rucker, AL

2:25 Effect of Prophylactic Naps and Caffeine on Alertness During Sleep Loss and Nocturnal Work Periods
Dr. Michael Bonnet, Dayton Department of Veteran Affairs Medical Center, Dayton, OH

3:00 DISCUSSION

3:30 Summary and Closing Remarks
Dr. John Vanderveen, Chair, Committee on Military Nutrition Research

4:00 ADJOURN

Workshop Abstracts

The abstracts appear in the order in which they were presented during the workshop on "Caffeine Formulations for Sustainment of Mental Task Performance During Military Operations," which was held on February 2–3, 1999, in Washington, D.C.

GENERAL OVERVIEW OF MILITARY INTEREST AND RESEARCH ON ROLE OF CAFFEINE IN PHYSICAL AND COGNITIVE PERFORMANCE

David Penetar, Ph.D.
U.S. Army Research Institute of Environmental Medicine, Natick, MA

The military's interest in caffeine is manifold and revolves around some of caffeine's basic behavioral effects: those of enhancing alertness, improving cognitive performance, and increasing physical capabilities. The degree and extent to which caffeine is an effective agent for producing these changes, especially with regard to the stressful, severe, and at times life-threatening environments in which military personnel operate, is a complex area for psychopharmacological research. Modern warfare pushes the limits of human performance in many ways. Military operations can have severe disrupting effects on normal sleep patterns and contain periods of sustained high rates of work and carrying of heavy loads. This disrupted sleep coupled with heavy physical demands can affect critical decision making and other cognitive skills. Under certain circumstances, pharmacological interventions may be warranted to prevent cognitive decrements as well as, possibly, the enhancement of physical performance. Several avenues of research have been pursued. The most notable effects of restricted and fragmented sleep are on alertness, mood, and cognitive abilities. Caffeine and other stimulants have been studied in both laboratory and field settings. These studies explore the effective dose range and time course of action. The use of caffeine to enhance physical performance in extreme environments (e.g., high altitude) or under high workload is also an area of military interest. The question of enhancing cognitive performance beyond the normal well-rested state is not yet completely answered. Continued research will contribute to policies outlining the acceptability and usefulness of caffeine in military operations.

CAFFEINE AND MUSCLE METABOLISM DURING PROLONGED EXERCISE

Lawrence L. Spriet, Ph.D.
Human Biology and Nutritional Science, University of Guelph, Ontario, Canada

Caffeine is a dietary pharmacological agent that is routinely ingested by people worldwide. It rapidly appears in the blood following ingestion, is taken up by the tissues of the body, and therefore has the potential to significantly alter metabolism. Many athletes also routinely ingest caffeine and there has been considerable interest in the ability of caffeine to enhance performance during prolonged aerobic exercise (Spriet, 1995). Several, well-controlled studies have established that moderate doses of caffeine (3–6 mg/kg body mass, about 2–4, 8-oz cups of coffee) ingested 1 hour prior to exercise enhance endurance performance in the laboratory at intensities of 70–85 percent of maximal oxygen uptake VO_{2max} (Costill et al., 1978; Graham and Spriet, 1995; Ivy et al., 1979; Pasman et al., 1995). Moderate caffeine doses produce urinary caffeine levels well below the allowable limit set by sports governing bodies (12 µg/mL), meaning that athletes can legally enhance their performance in this manner. Higher doses of caffeine (9–13 mg/kg body mass) also produce increases in laboratory endurance performance but are often associated with "illegal" urinary caffeine levels (> 12 µg/mL) and a higher incidence of adverse side effects (Graham and Sphet, 1991; Pasman et al., 1995; Spriet et al., 1992). The performance results are specific to well-trained elite or recreational athletes. These studies also demonstrate a large variability between individuals in the metabolic and performance responses to caffeine. Lastly, it is not known if these findings improve performance in competitions because controlled caffeine field studies are lacking.

The precise mechanisms responsible for improved performance during prolonged exercise remain elusive. A central nervous system contribution to the improved performance is always a possibility when studying humans, since it is not possible to separate the "central" and "peripheral" (skeletal muscle) effects of caffeine. However, it does appear that metabolic mechanisms are part of the explanation for the improvement in endurance performance following caffeine ingestion (5–13 mg/kg), except at low caffeine doses (2–4 mg/kg) where this has not been fully examined. The decreased respiratory exchange ratio, increased concentration of plasma-free fatty acids (FFAs) at the onset of exercise, glycogen sparing in the initial 15 minutes of exercise, and increased intramuscular triacylglycerol use during the first 30 minutes of exercise suggest a greater role for fat metabolism early in exercise following caffeine ingestion (Chesley et al., 1998; Essig et al., 1980; Graham and Spriet, 1991; Ivy et al., 1979; Spriet et al., 1992).

It has been suggested that the increased fat oxidation and decreased glycogen use in muscle following caffeine ingestion could be explained by the classic glucose–fatty acid cycle. In this scheme, elevated FFA availability to the muscle produced increases in muscle citrate and acetyl-coenzyme A, that were believed to inhibit the enzymes phosphofructokinase and pyruvate dehydrogenase. The subsequent decrease in glycolytic activity increased glucose 6-phosphate content, leading to inhibition of hexokinase and ultimately decreased muscle glucose uptake and oxidation. However, these mechanisms were not involved in the glycogen sparing during exercise at approximately 85 percent VO_{2max} with caffeine ingestion (Spriet et al., 1992). Instead, the mechanism for muscle glycogen sparing following caffeine ingestion appeared related to the regulation of glycogen phosphate activity via a more "defended" energy status of the cell. Subjects who spared muscle glycogen used less muscle phosphocreatine and had smaller increases in free adenosine 5'-monophosphate (AMP) and inorganic phosphate during exercise in the caffeine versus placebo trials (Chesley et al., 1998). The lower inorganic phosphate and AMP concentrations decreased the flux through glycogen phosphorylase and decreased glycogen use. There were no differences in these metabolites between trials in subjects who did not spare muscle glycogen. Presently, it is not clear how caffeine defends the energy state of the cell, but it may be related to an increased availability of fat and reducing equivalents (reduced nicotinamide–adenine dinucleotide) in the mitochondria at the onset of exercise.

Therefore, while it is clear that metabolic changes contribute to the ergogenic effect of caffeine during endurance exercise, aspects of the metabolic contribution have not been adequately examined in all situations. Measurements of muscle glycogen and triacylglycerol use and plasma FFA turnover are required to determine the magnitude of the metabolic link to improved performance at all caffeine doses and endurance exercise situations.

EFFECT OF CAFFEINE ON COGNITIVE FUNCTION AND ALERTNESS

Harris R. Lieberman, Ph.D.
U.S. Army Research Institute of Environmental Medicine, Natick, MA

Although the behavioral effects of caffeine have been a subject of scientific investigation for more than 100 years, it was not until recently that a clear picture of the substance's effects have started to emerge. Caffeine's effects on cognitive function and mood can be detected in rested and sleep-deprived volunteers using a variety of standardized tests. Only certain behavioral functions appear to be susceptible to the influence of moderate doses of caffeine. In particular, it appears that in well-rested volunteers, low and moderate doses of caffeine (32–256 mg) preferentially affect functions related to vigilance—the ability of individuals to maintain alertness and appropriate responsiveness to the external environment for sustained periods of time. Self-reported mood states that are related to vigilance, such as alertness, also are clearly improved by moderate doses of caffeine. Higher cognitive functions, such as memory and visuospatial reasoning, do not appear to be affected in any substantial manner when the substance is administered in moderate doses to rested volunteers.

Among individuals who have been deprived of sleep, vigilance tests and mood questionnaires remain highly sensitive to the beneficial effects of caffeine. In addition, certain more complex cognitive functions also improve, although these effects may be secondary to improved vigilance. Recently we conducted a field study that demonstrated that even when volunteers are exposed to severe sleep deprivation in combination with mental, physical, and psychological stress, moderate doses of caffeine can partially restore vigilance and other key aspects of cognitive performance. This study may provide useful insight into the optimal dose of caffeine to employ under such circumstances.

Maintenance of vigilance is critical for a variety of military duties such as standing watch, sentry duty, communication monitoring, and operating vehicles, including aircraft and vessels. During military operations a single individual can be responsible for the safety of hundreds of individuals traveling in his or her vehicle or being protected by his or her weapons system. Therefore, lapses in vigilance can have devastating consequences. Even in well-rested individuals vigilance significantly deteriorates after brief periods of attempting to maintain optimal alertness during boring but critical activities. During wartime or other intense operations, sleep loss and environmental and psychological stress greatly reduce the ability of individuals to maintain even marginally adequate vigilance. Therefore, administration of caffeine in appropriate doses at the correct times may be an effective method for substantially improving key aspects of cognitive function in rested and sleep-deprived war fighters.

CAFFEINE AND SENTRY DUTY PERFORMANCE

Richard F. Johnson, Ph.D.
U.S. Army Research Institute of Environmental Medicine, Natick, MA

Proficient sentry duty performance requires both rifle marksmanship accuracy and sufficient alertness to detect the infrequent appearance of targets. At the U.S. Army Research Institute of Environmental Medicine, the Weaponeer M16 Rifle Marksmanship Simulator, a U.S. Army training device, has been adapted for assessing the components of sentry duty (target detection and rifle firing accuracy). Our research has shown that during 3 hours of baseline sentry duty, the soldier's speed of target detection becomes slower while rifle firing accuracy remains unimpaired.

In our first caffeine study with the sentry duty model, we tested the effects of the ingestion of 200 mg of caffeine on male soldiers' target detection speed and rifle firing accuracy. Target detection speed under the placebo condition deteriorated with time and was significantly slower after 60–90 minutes on the task. Under the caffeine condition, the impairment in target detection speed was significantly attenuated. Regardless of drug condition, rifle firing accuracy showed no impairment during sentry duty.

Our second caffeine study was sponsored by the Defense Women's Health Research Program and focused on the sentry duty performance of both men and women. Both men's and women's target detection speeds deteriorated with time on sentry duty, and this performance decrement was eliminated by 200 mg of caffeine. While men's rifle-firing accuracy remained constant over time, women's rifle firing accuracy deteriorated after 90 minutes, regardless of drug condition.

Our third caffeine study, recently completed, was a replication and extension of the second and introduced the requirement to discriminate friendly from enemy targets. The decrement in both men's and women's target detection speed with time on sentry duty was again eliminated by 200 mg of caffeine. As in the second study, women's rifle firing accuracy was poorer than that of men's, but the relationship with time on the task was complex and did not clearly replicate the results of the second study. Compared to placebo, the number of correct target identifications (friend versus foe) was significantly improved by 200 mg of caffeine.

Conclusions

1. *Efficacy:* Without impairing rifle-firing accuracy, 200 mg of caffeine improves target detection speed and increases the likelihood of correct friend–foe target identifications during simulated sentry duty.

2. *Safety:* No adverse effects of caffeine were observed during these studies.

3. *Dose:* In sentry duty, effects of caffeine in doses other than that used in these studies (200 mg) is unknown.

4. *Alternatives:* Sentry duty of less than 60 minutes' duration does not lead to a decrement in performance and would not benefit from the prior ingestion of caffeine.

5. *Formulation:* We have tested caffeine only in the 200-mg tablet form.

EYELID MOVEMENT AS A PHYSIOLOGICAL PREDICTOR OF COGNITIVE IMPAIRMENT DURING SLEEP DEPRIVATION

Robert Stickgold, Ph.D.
Department of Psychiatry, Harvard Medical School, Boston, MA

Overall cognitive performance is modulated during sleep deprivation by both homeostatic and circadian factors. However, on a shorter time scale, performance decrements can be reversed by heightened interest and attention on the part of the subject. Within this context, it would be valuable to be able to easily monitor levels of functional arousal using physiological rather than behavioral measures. From a theoretical perspective, this would allow clarification of the role of attention and arousal in the maintenance of performance on specific tasks. From a more practical perspective, it could allow the ongoing monitoring and predicting of performance level before and during the execution of critical tasks.

We have developed a home-based sleep and vigilance monitor called the "Nightcap". The Nightcap uses a piezoelectric film to monitor both tonic and phasic muscle activity in the upper eyelid and has been used during waking and sleep, including periods of sleep deprivation. Activity is quantified as the number of 250-ms epochs/minute in which eyelid movement exceeds a threshold amount. This activity not only identifies sleep onset with high reliability but, in pilot studies, also correlates with levels of performance on a series of cognitive tests during periods of sleep deprivation.

In a pilot study, performance on a vigilance test administered repeatedly over 40 hours of sleep deprivation varied dramatically as a function of both homeostatic and circadian factors and correlated highly with eyelid activity recorded during the tests, measured both as reaction times (Pearson r-value = -0.82, df = 8, $p < 0.005$) and as error rates (Pearson r-value = -0.80, df = 8, $p < 0.005$). Overall, eyelid activity explained two-thirds of the variance in performance.

In contrast, performance on a mental rotation task was not diminished during sleep deprivation, with both reaction time and accuracy showing nonsignificant improvement with increased deprivation. Eyelid activity also showed no sleep deprivation effect during the mental rotation tests, despite the strong variations measured over the same 40 hours during the vigilance tests.

We conclude that the eyelid activity measured by the Nightcap reflects instantaneous arousal levels that correlate at the behavioral level with task performance on a range of cognitive tests. We believe that this eyelid activity reflects the modulatory activity of brainstem arousal systems that control both levels of behavioral arousal and the levator palpebrae muscle of the upper eyelid. As a result, the eyelid sensor permits both the monitoring of brainstem arousal systems and the prediction of behavioral outcomes.

CIRCADIAN AND SLEEP HOMEOSTATIC MODULATION OF SLEEP AND PERFORMANCE

James K. Wyatt, Ph.D.
Harvard Medical School and Brigham and Women's Hospital, Boston, MA

Two processes that contribute significantly to the modulation of sleep and waking neurobehavioral functioning are the sleep homeostat and the endogenous circadian pacemaker. Although the exact neurophysiological and neuropharmacological mechanisms remain to be conclusively delineated, the sleep homeostatic process can be found in impairments of neurobehavioral functioning with increasing durations of sustained wakefulness. Thus, minimal sleep homeostatic impairment of alertness and performance is seen during the first few hours of wakefulness and increases thereafter. In its modulation of sleep continuity and structure, maximal sleep pressure is seen during the first third of a typical 8-hour sleep episode, with very low homeostatic drive for sleep in the final third.

In contrast, the endogenous circadian pacemaker, located in the suprachiasmatic nucleus of the hypothalamus, has a paradoxical phase relationship with the sleep homeostatic process. This relationship is beneficial, and in fact critical, in maintaining relatively stable alertness and performance across a typical, daytime, 16-hour wake episode. This is due to the higher homeostatic drive for sleep being offset by the maximal circadian drive for wakefulness in the latter half of the habitual waking day. Similarly, the low homeostatic drive for sleep seen during the latter part of the habitual sleep episode is offset by the circadian drive for sleep, which is itself maximal 1–2 hours prior to habitual wake time.

Under conditions of challenge to the sleep homeostatic system (e.g., sustained wakefulness of extended duty hours) and/or the circadian system (e.g., jet lag or night operations), impairments of neurobehavioral functioning become impressively evident. In our laboratory experiments with healthy normal volunteers, we have simulated exposure to rapid time-zone travel (bedtimes and wake times shifting) and extended duty hours (28.57-hour wake episodes and 14.28-hour sleep episodes) with a month-long protocol. Though blind to drug condition at this point, at the end of this study we hope to have information on the efficacy of low-dose, sustained caffeine administration as a countermeasure to deficits of neurobehavioral functioning encountered during this type of biological challenge.

Preliminary data are presented demonstrating the relative strength of homeostatic and circadian modulation of sleep propensity, sleep structure, and sleep consolidation seen under these conditions. Data are presented on the homeostatic and circadian modulation of several neurobehavioral measures, including reaction time and visual vigilance, short-term memory, cognitive throughput, and subjective alertness.

CAFFEINE EFFECTS DURING SLEEP DEPRIVATION AND RECOVERY

George Bray, M.D., Harris Lieberman, Ph.D., Richard Magill, Ph.D., Donna Ryan, M.D., Steve Smith, M.D., Julia Volaufova, and William Waters
Pennington Biomedical Research Center and Louisiana State University, Baton Rouge, LA

Objective

The objective of this study was to determine the effectiveness of central nervous system-activating substances (d-amphetamine, caffeine, phentermine, tyrosine), compared to placebo, on the following parameters during sleep deprivation and recovery: (1) sleep drive, (2) sleep quantity, (3) sleep quality, (4) mental and fine motor performance, and (5) biochemistry of the pituitary–adrenal axis.

Methods

To accomplish this task, we recruited 76 healthy males, ages 18–35, body mass index 20–27 kg/m^2, who participated in a parallel arm, randomized, double-blind, placebo-controlled study comparing tyrosine 150 mg/kg body weight (BW), phentermine 37.5 mg, d-amphetamine 20 mg, or caffeine 300 mg/70 kg BW, to placebo. We performed multiple polysomnography recordings, cognitive performance tests, and neuroendocrine assays before and during 40 hours of sleep deprivation and also during a recovery night.

Results

In sleep-deprived adults, we found a significant delay in time to sleep onset for amphetamine, compared to placebo. The amphetamine effect persisted longer than caffeine and phentermine. Caffeine significantly delays sleep onset compared to placebo, but not as greatly as amphetamine. Time to sleep onset latency was significantly greater for amphetamine and phentermine compared to placebo at recovery night. Caffeine did not appear to interfere with time to sleep onset during recovery. Amphetamine significantly decreased sleep quantity (decreased total sleep time, decreased sleep efficiency, increased sleep onset latency, increased wakefulness after sleep onset) whereas caffeine had an effect on sleep quantity during recovery similar to placebo. Amphetamine and phentermine significantly impaired sleep depth during recovery (decrease in percentage of rapid eye movement [REM], increased latency to REM). Amphetamine and phentermine produced significantly more awakenings than other agents tested. Caffeine had a profile similar to placebo (and tyrosine) in terms of sleep depth, architecture, and continuity during recovery. Amphetamine, caffeine, and phentermine significantly improved most target performance measures that show a performance decrement during sleep deprivation (logical reasoning, running memory, math processing, pursuit tracking, visual vigilance). Performance decrements during sleep deprivation were chiefly in response time and improvements were in response time, without sacrifices in accuracy.

Conclusions

The model demonstrated that caffeine is effective in reversing the negative effects on alertness during sleep deprivation. This effect was similar to phentermine, significantly better than placebo, but less than the observed effects of amphetamine. In contrast to amphetamine and phentermine, caffeine had no deleterious effects on recovery sleep. Caffeine, amphetamine, and phentermine all had significant beneficial effects on performance indicators during sleep deprivation, especially with regard to response time. Caffeine is a candidate for policy implementation in conditions where sleep deprivation is inevitable. Furthermore, we suggest that future studies be conducted in situations that mimic military duty conditions in order to confirm these findings.

CIRCADIAN AND HOMEOSTATIC INTERACTIONS IN WAKING NEUROBEHAVIORAL FUNCTIONS DURING PARTIAL AND TOTAL SLEEP DEPRIVATION: EFFECTS OF CAFFEINE

Hans P.A. Van Dongen, Ph.D. and David F. Dinges, Ph.D.
Unit for Experimental Psychiatry, University of Pennsylvania School of Medicine, Supported by AFOSR grant F49620-95-1-0388, and IEPRF

This ongoing double-blind, placebo-controlled, randomized trial of low-dose caffeine simulates the effects of sustained operations with and without sleep and caffeine, on a total of 56 male adults in the controlled environment of an isolated laboratory with light not brighter than 50 lux (range 25–45 lux). On 3 subsequent baseline days, subjects have 8 hours time for sleep (from 2330 until 0730 hours). During the next 3 days in the laboratory (i.e., 88 hours), they are either partially sleep-deprived (PSD) or totally sleep-deprived (TSD), In the PSD condition, 2-hour naps are taken every 12 hours, that is, from 1445 until 1645 hours and from 0245 until 0445 hours. During this 88-hour period of sleep deprivation, neurobehavioral tests are performed every 2 hours, waking electroencephalogram and sleep polysomnography with additional EEG and rectal temperature measurements are recorded continuously, and blood samples are taken every 90 minutes for the analysis of cortisol, melatonin, catecholamines, and plasma caffeine.

In this trial, there are 4 groups of 14 subjects each: TSD + sustained low-dose caffeine, TSD + placebo, PSD + sustained low-dose caffeine, and PSD + placebo. Starting at 0530 hours of sleep deprivation day one, subjects in the caffeine conditions receive a 0.3-mg/kg caffeine pill each hour, and the remaining subjects receive a placebo pill each hour (except when napping in the PSD condition). As of yet, the investigators are still blinded to conditions. Therefore, no results of the efficacy of caffeine intake on reducing neurobehavioral performance deficits in this protocol can be reported. In body temperature and plasma melatonin, however, a circadian phase delay is observed during sleep deprivation, regardless of deprivation condition (PSD or TSD). Clearly, since the investigators are still blinded, the involvement of caffeine in this phase drift cannot be determined, but the finding of Redman and Rajaratnam (1998) that caffeine induces a circadian phase advance in rats makes it unlikely that caffeine would cause the presently observed phase delay in humans.

CAFFEINE RESEARCH IN THE NAVY

W.K. Prusaczyk, Ph.D.
Naval Health Research Center, San Diego, CA

Navy policy precludes stocking or using amphetamines or sedatives to maintain or enhance performance. Due to their widespread acceptance and relative safety, caffeine and nicotine are frequently used to combat the effects of fatigue during sustained military operations. In fact, the Naval Aerospace and Operational Medical Institute has disseminated protocols for use of these products. With the Navy's current emphasis on a smoke- and nicotine-free fleet, the interest in caffeine is increasing. During Operation Southern Watch over Iraq, among carrier-based aircrew, caffeine was the preferred modality for maintenance of performance. Belland and Bissell (1993) reported that 63 percent of aircrew surveyed used some form of nonpharmaceutical stimulant. Of these, 75 percent used caffeine either as coffee (1–7 cups preflight) or caffeine tablets to maintain performance during the sustained operations.

Caffeine research in the Navy has, as do most areas of pharmacological performance enhancement research, two thrusts—physiological and psychological. In a study of the effects of caffeine on thermoregulatory responses, Ahlers et al. (1990) found that caffeine (3.5 mg/kg^{-1}) significantly attenuated rectal temperature afterdrop following cold water immersion. Subjects had an induced $0.5°C$ rectal temperature. At the nadir of afterdrop, subjects taking caffeine had a $0.3°C$ higher mean rectal temperature and returned to preafterdrop temperature sooner.

Caffeine has a purported ergogenic effect of sparing muscle glycogen. Prusaczyk et al. (1998) investigated the effect of caffeine on reducing muscle glycogen use following a carbohydrate loading protocol. In this double-blind, placebo-controlled study, it was found that caffeine did not alter the rate of glycogen use during prolonged exercise in carbohydrate-loaded subjects.

Studies of the psychological effects of caffeine ingestion have focused on the alleviation of fatigue and maintenance of mood during periods of sustained or continuous operations and during sleep deprivation. In 1995, Bonnet et al. reported the effects of prophylactic naps (0, 2, 4, or 8 hours) or caffeine (0, 150, 300, or 400 mg) on performance (logical reasoning, hand tremor, digit symbol substitution task) during 52 hours of sleep deprivation. The long nap was better than caffeine for maintaining performance, mood, and alertness. A repeated low dose of caffeine was better than no nap or large single doses of caffeine; however, neither nap nor caffeine could preserve performance at baseline levels beyond 24 hours.

Kelly et al. (1996, 1997) examined the effects of caffeine dosing (300 mg every 6 hours, 400 mg and placebo alternated every 6 hours, and placebo every 6 hours) during 64 hours of sleep deprivation on subsequent recovery sleep. Polysomnography revealed that caffeine affected sleep only during the first third of the first recovery night. Compared to baseline, caffeine-ingesting subjects showed lighter Stage 2 sleep and decreased slow wave sleep. Caffeine may, in fact, make short sleeps deeper if not ingested close to sleep. The authors concluded that repeated caffeine dosing during deprivation appears not to interfere with recovery sleep following sleep deprivation.

CAFFEINE AS A MODEL DRUG OF ABUSE

Stephen G. Holtzman, Ph.D.
Department of Pharmacology, Emory University School of Medicine, Atlanta, GA

Low to moderate doses of caffeine produce many effects in humans and animals that resemble effects produced by low doses of nonxanthine psychomotor stimulants, such as amphetamine and cocaine. For example, they produce positive mood states and increases in wakefulness and motor activity. This has given rise to the inevitable question of whether or not caffeine has abuse liability. In fact, caffeine does have the principal features usually associated with a drug of abuse. These will be reviewed, drawing largely from studies in the preclinical literature and, where appropriate, will be compared to those of nonxanthine psychomotor stimulants.

Caffeine is reinforcing; humans and animals will work to get it, albeit not as hard as they will work to get other stimulant drugs. Caffeine is discriminable; humans and animals can recognize the fact that they have received caffeine. The discriminative effects of low to moderate doses of caffeine have commonalities with those of nonxanthine stimulants. Chronic administration of caffeine results in the development of insurmountable drug-specific tolerance to many effects, including psychomotor stimulation, as well as in physical dependence. The latter state is characterized by a subjective withdrawal syndrome in humans that includes headache, lethargy, and difficulty concentrating and by reduced activity in animals when caffeine administration is stopped.

The catecholamine neurotransmitters norepinephrine and dopamine have a prominent role in the autonomic and behavioral effects of nonxanthine stimulants. In animals, brain dopamine, in particular, has been implicated in the psychomotor stimulant effects of these drugs and in other actions relevant to potential for abuse, such as discriminative stimulus and reinforcing stimulus effects. Caffeine also enhances neurotransmission mediated by dopamine. However, in contrast to amphetamine and cocaine, which dramatically increase the concentration of dopamine in the synapse, the effects of caffeine on brain dopamine are more subtle and modest. The effects are secondary to the blockade of adenosine receptors by caffeine and are not associated with elevated concentrations of dopamine in the synapse.

Moderate to high doses of caffeine produce behavioral effects that are different from those produced by lower doses of caffeine and by nonxanthine psychomotor stimulants. They often produce negative mood states in humans, with anxiety a prominent component, and appear to be aversive to animals. There is no evidence of tolerance to these effects. The neural mechanisms that underlie the high-dose effects of caffeine remain obscure.

It is evident that caffeine has most of the features of a drug of abuse. Nevertheless, the abuse liability of caffeine is negligible in comparison to that of many nonxanthine psychomotor stimulants. The reasons for this include the less intense psychomotor stimulant effects of low to moderate doses, the development of tolerance to those effects, and the often unpleasant and persistent effects of high doses that serve to limit drug intake by many individuals.

CAFFEINE PHYSICAL DEPENDENCE AND THE CONSEQUENCES OF CAFFEINE ABSTINENCE

Roland R. Griffiths, Ph.D.
Department of Psychiatry and Neuroscience, Behavioral Biology Research Center, Johns Hopkins University School of Medicine, Baltimore, MD

Physical dependence is manifested by time-limited biochemical, physiological, and behavioral disruptions (i.e., a withdrawal syndrome) upon termination of chronic or repeated drug administration. There have been more than 10 reports of caffeine withdrawal in laboratory animals, most of which have documented substantial behavioral disruptions following cessation of chronic caffeine dosing (e.g., 50–80 percent reductions in spontaneous locomotor activity; 20–50 percent reductions in operant responding). These studies have examined caffeine withdrawal in rats, cats, and monkeys.

Caffeine physical dependence has been clearly demonstrated in humans in approximately 60 case reports and human experimental studies. The most frequently reported withdrawal symptom is headache (also cerebral fullness), which is characterized as being gradual in development, diffuse, throbbing, and sometimes severe. Other symptoms, in roughly decreasing order of prominence, are drowsiness (e.g., increased sleepiness and yawning, decreased energy and alertness); increased work difficulty (decreased motivation for tasks or work, impaired concentration); decreased feelings of well-being or contentment (decreased self-confidence, increased irritability); decreased sociability, friendliness, or talkativeness; flu-like feelings (muscle aches or stiffness, hot or cold spells, heavy feelings in arms or legs, nausea); and blurred vision. In addition to these symptoms, composite scales of depression and anxiety may be elevated and psychomotor performance may be impaired. The occurrence of headache as a withdrawal symptom does not necessarily correlate with the occurrence of other symptoms (e.g., tiredness), suggesting that other signs and symptoms are not merely epiphenomena of headache.

The severity of caffeine withdrawal is an increasing function of caffeine maintenance dose. When symptoms of caffeine withdrawal occur, the severity can vary from mild to extreme. At its worst, caffeine withdrawal is incompatible with normal functioning and is sometimes totally incapacitating.

The incidence of caffeine withdrawal is an increasing function of caffeine maintenance dose. The best estimates of the incidence of caffeine withdrawal in the general population come from a survey study and an experimental study. A recent random-digit dial telephone survey in Vermont showed that among current users of caffeine who reported that they had abstained from caffeine for 24 hours or more, 27 percent reported withdrawal headaches when they abstained. The experimental study involved 62 individuals from the general community with a distribution of caffeine intake similar to the general population in the United States (mean caffeine intake of 235 mg). The study involved a double-blind, approximately 48-hour, caffeine abstinence trial under conditions that obscured the fact that the purpose of the study was to investigate caffeine. During caffeine withdrawal 52 percent reported moderate or severe headache and 8–11 percent showed abnormally high scores on standardized depression, anxiety, and fatigue scales. The incidence of headache observed from the survey and experimental study in the general population (27–52 percent) is in the range of that observed in several other recent studies conducted in special subject populations.

Although the incidence and severity of caffeine withdrawal are an increasing function of caffeine dose, two studies have shown that caffeine withdrawal can occur after relatively long-term administration of caffeine doses as low as 100 mg.

The caffeine withdrawal syndrome follows an orderly time course. Onset has usually been reported to occur 12–24 hours after terminating caffeine intake, although onset as late as 36 hours has been documented. Peak withdrawal intensity has generally been described as occurring 20–48 hours after abstinence. The duration of caffeine withdrawal has most often been described as ranging between 2 days and 1 week, although longer durations have been noted occasionally.

Physiological mechanisms underlying caffeine withdrawal remain uncertain, although some studies suggest that increased blood volume, possibly adenosine-mediated, may be involved with caffeine withdrawal headache.

Implications of Caffeine Physical Dependence for Performance Assessment

In assessing the effects of caffeine on performance, many previous studies have failed to differentiate between caffeine's restoring performance degraded by caffeine abstinence versus caffeine's enhancing performance. In examining such studies, attention should be given to the habitual daily caffeine dose consumed by subjects and the duration of caffeine abstinence immediately before testing. The effects of caffeine on performance may depend on a given individual's level of caffeine tolerance (decreased responsiveness to the drug due to repeated past exposure) and physical dependence (behavioral disruptions upon termination of repeated drug administration).

POSITIVE EFFECTS OF CAFFEINE OR NEGATIVE EFFECTS OF CAFFEINE WITHDRAWAL

Andrew Smith, Ph.D., and G.H. Rubin
Health Psychology Research Unit, Department of Experimental Psychology
University of Bristol, United Kingdom

This paper will consider the extent to which differences between caffeinated and decaffeinated conditions reflect the positive effects of caffeine or the negative effects of caffeine withdrawal. The background to this debate is presented and the relevant literature reviewed. It is concluded that the absence of strong negative effects of caffeine withdrawal on performance, and the demonstration of positive effects in nonconsumers, support the view that caffeine enhances performance and does not just remove impairments induced by withdrawal.

The second part of the paper will consider in detail the health consequences of withdrawal. Results on headaches and caffeine withdrawal will be discussed and it will be concluded that the increased incidence of headaches following caffeine withdrawal reflects factors such as expectancies and the ability to determine whether the caffeine has been withdrawn or not. This view will be contrasted with those suggesting a pharmacological addiction to caffeine.

Abstract

Previous research has shown that cessation of caffeine consumption may be associated with a distinct withdrawal syndrome, typified by an increase in headaches. Recent research suggests that low to moderate consumers of caffeine may report an increase in headaches if they perceive caffeine to have been withdrawn regardless of whether it has been or not. The present study provides additional support for the role of subjective perceptions in the caffeine withdrawal syndrome. Forty-four low-caffeine consumers recorded the incidence of headaches when drinking caffeinated or decaffeinated beverages. When caffeine was withdrawn the incidence of headaches increased, but this effect was significant only in those individuals who could discriminate whether they were consuming caffeinated or decaffeinated beverages. This result suggests a major role of subjective perceptions and expectancies in the caffeine withdrawal syndrome, a view that contrasts the notion that a significant proportion of caffeine consumers are physically dependent upon caffeine.

APPENDIX A

Introduction

A number of studies have demonstrated that cessation of caffeine consumption may result in a distinct withdrawal syndrome, typified by the occurrence of headaches (Dreisbach and Pfeiffer, 1943; Griffiths et al., 1990; Strain et al., 1994; van Dusseldorp and Katan, 1990). In the light of this evidence, caffeine withdrawal syndrome has been included in DSM-IV. These studies have tended to use individuals with histories of chronic high-dose caffeine consumption (≥ 500 mg) or else have increased the caffeine intake of participants to very high levels during the caffeinated condition of the experiment itself. Even with high-caffeine consumers the proportion of participants who report headaches during withdrawal has ranged from 25 to 100 percent. Similarly, those studies that have investigated withdrawal in low-dose consumers (< 200 mg) have found that headache reporting varies from 20 percent of the sample (Fennelly et al., 1991) to 50 percent (Silverman et al., 1992) or even 100 percent (Naismith et al., 1970)

Results from a recent study (Smith, 1996) suggest that low- to moderate-caffeine consumers may report an increase in headaches when they perceive caffeine to have been withdrawn regardless of whether it has been or not. The reporting of headache is seen, therefore, as a combination of an expectancy that caffeine withdrawal may increase headaches and the ability to discriminate whether caffeine has actually been withdrawn. This view is very different from previous assertions that a significant proportion of low- to moderate-caffeine consumers are physically dependent upon caffeine. Support for the role of subjective perceptions comes from our latest study of this issue, which is described below.

Method

Participants

Forty-three regular caffeinated tea and coffee consumers (22 females, 21 males, mean age 21.1 years, range 18–26 years) participated in a study examining the effects of caffeine withdrawal on reporting of headaches. Mean reported daily caffeine consumption from these sources was 175 mg (standard deviation = 91 mg; based on caffeine content of products provided by Debry [1994]). Each volunteer carried out a 2-day baseline period during which normal caffeine consumption was recorded using a diary, and headaches and other symptoms were measured. For all volunteers, either tea or coffee was the major source of caffeine. Following this the volunteers were given supplies of either caffeinated or decaffeinated tea and coffee and told to continue with their normal pattern of consumption but to use only the coffee and tea supplied. Volunteers were blind with regard to which days they were given decaffeinated products or caffeinated products. They were told to stop their normal consumption of other caffeinated products such as chocolates or soft drinks. Each volunteer carried out both caffeinated and decaffeinated conditions for 2 days, the order of conditions being counterbalanced across participants. In addition to recording the presence or absence of headache and other symptoms, volunteers were asked whether they believed the beverages consumed that day to have been caffeinated or decaffeinated.

Results

The results showed that there was no significant difference in reporting headaches in the baseline (14.0 percent of sample reported a headache) and caffeinated drink conditions (18.6 percent). However, when caffeine was withdrawn, the frequency of headache increased to 39.5 percent (significantly greater than both baseline and caffeinated conditions, $p < 0.01$). Further analyses revealed that the effect of caffeine withdrawal depended on whether the participants were able to discriminate whether caffeine was present or not (22 participants correctly identified the two conditions). An analysis of variance showed that the condition x ability to discriminate caffeine was significant ($F(2, 78) = 4.29, p < 0.05$). For those who could tell whether caffeine was withdrawn or not, headache frequency increased from 7 percent in the baseline and 9.3 percent in the caffeinated condition to 48.8 percent in the decaffeinated condition. In contrast to this, caffeine withdrawal had little effect on headache reporting in those unable to tell the nature of the beverages (see Figure 1). Overall, the observed effect of caffeine withdrawal on headache frequency appeared to be due entirely to the reporting of headaches by those participants who were able to correctly identify whether caffeinated or decaffeinated drinks were consumed.

Discussion

Three possible explanations exist to explain the link between reporting of headaches and ability to discriminate whether or not the drinks were caffeinated. First, some individuals may develop headaches during caffeine withdrawal and use the increased symptoms to help identify the nature of the drinks. Alternatively, those individuals who could identify the nature of the drinks would then be influenced by the expectancy that caffeine withdrawal increases headache frequency. In contrast, those unable to discriminate between caffeinated and decaffeinated conditions would show no difference in headache frequency in these two conditions but should report an increase relative to baseline. This was found here. Finally, it is possible that both mechanisms may be involved in the overall pattern of results. In this context, one can view the expectancy effect as a factor that has inflated estimates of the number of people who are dependent on caffeine rather than being a total explanation for the caffeine withdrawal–headache association. Studies of headaches in patients withdrawn from caffeine prior to surgery suggest that headache frequency is around 25 percent. Given that

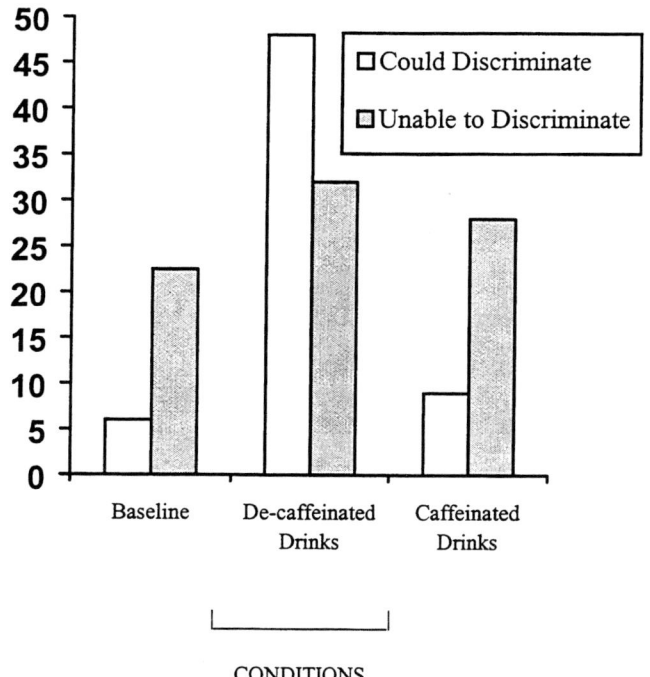

FIGURE 1 Percentage of volunteers reporting headaches in the various conditions (those who correctly identified the caffeine versus those who could not).

baseline headache rate in nonwithdrawn volunteers studied here was nearly 15 percent, one can see that we are clearly not looking at a large effect. Indeed, it may be that individuals who regularly get a lot of headaches do not show an increase when caffeine is withdrawn and are also poor at discriminating whether they have been consuming caffeinated beverages or not. Further research is required to resolve this issue.

Conclusion

In conclusion, the present study has demonstrated that the increased frequency of headaches during caffeine withdrawal reflects participants' detecting they are in that condition and reporting the symptoms they expect to be associated with it. Further research should address the direction of causality between perceptions of caffeine content and withdrawal symptoms. In addition, the extent to which similar effects are observed in those who consume higher doses of caffeine requires further investigation.

Acknowledgment

Professor Smith's caffeine research is supported by the Physiological Effects of Caffeine Research Fund of the Institute for Scientific Information on Coffee.

PHARMACOLOGY OF CAFFEINE

Gary H. Kamimori, Ph.D.
Department of Neurobiology and Behavior, Division of Neuropsychiatry, Walter Reed Army Institute of Research, Washington, DC

Caffeine is one of the most widely used drugs in the world. It is a naturally occurring stimulant that has a variety of unique characteristics. Although the pharmacokinetics and pharmacodynamics of caffeine have been the subject of thousands of studies over the past century, many of its characteristics (e.g., mechanisms of action, stimulant properties) are still unclear. The purpose of this presentation is to provide an overview of current knowledge pertaining to the pharmacokinetic characteristics, efficacy, safety, dynamic effects, and possible formulations for the delivery of caffeine. In addition, we review past and current caffeine research from the Department of Neurobiology and Behavior of the Walter Reed Army Institute of Research.

DESIGN OF A FOOD MATRIX FOR THE DELIVERY OF PERFORMANCE-ENHANCING COMPONENTS

Jack Briggs, M.S.
U.S. Army Soldier Biological Chemical Command, Natick Soldier Center, Natick, MA

The utilization of performance-enhancing agents has a two-fold approach. First, the efficacy of the agent must be established using physiological and/or cognitive measurements. Second, a delivery system is necessary that ensures timely availability of the agent to the physiological point of need. There are several delivery systems currently available: transdermal, pills (including time release), inhalants, injections, and incorporation of the agent into food. The mode of delivery for the military is incorporation into common foods and restriction of any performance agent to that of a natural food constituent such as proteins, amino acids, antioxidants, and caffeine. There are several considerations when incorporating performance-enhancing agents into foods:

1. compatibility of the agent with the other food components,
2. shelf-life stability,
3. physiological uptake and delivery of the agent to the target organs, and
4. acceptance of the food item to ensure consumption of nutrients in the fortified item.

The military shelf-life requirements of 3 years at 80°F and 6 months at 100°F make this even more challenging than commercially developed products, which have a shorter shelf life.

This paper focuses on the development of a chocolate–caffeine food bar and placebo to be used in physiological performance testing. The bar was designed to deliver 6 mg of caffeine per kg weight of the subject (i.e., a 75-g bar for a 105-kg subject would contain 632 mg of caffeine, equivalent to 6 cups of coffee). In order to mask this level of caffeine, a chocolate mocha-flavored bar matrix was chosen. The bar weight was adjusted to maintain consistent dose weight for variable subject weights. Caffeine is a very bitter ingredient, which creates food technological challenges in developing an acceptable product, as well as a placebo that looks and tastes like the product. The bars were fed to military subjects prior to physical training. Caffeine uptake and distribution were monitored over a 2-hour period by analysis of caffeine in the subject's saliva.

CAFFEINE AND CARBOHYDRATE SUPPLEMENTS FOR PHYSICAL PERFORMANCE

John L. Ivy, Ph.D.
Exercise and Metabolism Laboratory, Department of Kinesiology and Health Education, University of Texas, Austin

Both caffeine and carbohydrate supplementation have been found to have ergogenic effects on aerobic endurance and athletic performance. The means by which these supplements induce their ergogenic effects occur through different mechanisms of action and may be influenced by the type and intensity of exercise. There is ample evidence that caffeine improves aerobic endurance by increasing fat oxidation and sparing muscle. This is very beneficial for prolonged aerobic exercise in which muscle glycogen is a required fuel source. Caffeine also appears to function as a neurological stimulant and may improve aerobic endurance and exercise performance at high exercise intensities by reducing perception of effort and masking symptoms of fatigue. During prolonged low-intensity exercise, or prolonged exercise that varies from low to moderate intensity, carbohydrate supplementation improves aerobic endurance by increasing reliance on blood glucose and sparing muscle glycogen. When the exercise is moderately intense (65 to 75 percent, VO_{2max}), carbohydrate supplementation does not spare muscle glycogen but enhances aerobic endurance by preventing the onset of hypoglycemia and maintaining an adequate rate of carbohydrate oxidation. Because the ergogenic effects of caffeine and carbohydrate supplementation occur through different mechanisms of action, it can be theorized that their effects on endurance performance would be additive. However, carbohydrate supplementation blunts the exercise-induced increase in lipolysis and inhibits fat oxidation. Therefore, the ergogenic effect of caffeine may actually be blunted, rather than enhanced, by the addition of carbohydrate to a caffeine supplement. Whether the combination of caffeine and carbohydrate supplements functions additively or antagonistically may depend on the type and intensity of exercise being performed and the timing of the supplementation. These conditions are discussed with regard to the ergogenic effects of each supplement.

COGNITIVE PERFORMANCE EFFECTS OF CAFFEINE VERSUS AMPHETAMINE FOLLOWING SLEEP DEPRIVATION

Mary A. Kautz, Ph.D.
Department of Neurobiology and Behavior, Walter Reed Army Institute of Research, Washington, DC

With sustained military operations, round-the-clock work schedules often lead to sleep deprivation. It has been well documented that sleep deprivation impairs cognitive performance and alters mood, with a consequent increased threat to safety and productivity in a variety of industrial and military settings. Stimulants have long been used to reduce the effects of sleep loss and to counteract the sleepiness resulting from irregular work–rest hours. A number of studies in our laboratory at Walter Reed Army Institute of Research have examined the effects of stimulant administration following prolonged periods of wakefulness. Here, we present a comparison of the effects of caffeine and amphetamine in subjects who are tested through a total of 64 hours sleep deprivation. Performance, alertness, and mood measurements were taken throughout the study. At 48 hours of sleep deprivation, a dose of caffeine (150, 300, or 600 mg), amphetamine (5, 10, or 20 mg), or placebo was administered, and testing continued for at least 12 hours postdose. Both compounds, at the highest dose tested for each, produced comparable results in the following ways: cognitive performance improved and was sustained for 12 hours; measures of objective alertness improved; and there was an improvement in self-ratings of mood. There were also some adverse side effects, with amphetamine producing mild cardiovascular disturbances, disruptions in recovery sleep, and feelings of euphoria, while caffeine resulted in increased subjective reports of tremor and ratings of anxiety. Our recommendation is that given the universal availability and socially acceptable use of caffeine (with relatively few adverse side effects), it can be used only to "postpone" sleep up to 12 hours, not to replace it. Future studies in our laboratory will assess the synthetic compound modafinil, currently indicated for improving alertness in narcoleptics, and compare modafinil to caffeine and amphetamine in our standard paradigm of measuring cognitive performance, alertness, and mood.

USE OF AMPHETAMINE TO COUNTERACT SLEEP DEPRIVATION IN AVIATORS

John Caldwell, Ph.D.
Sustained Operations Research, U.S. Army Aeromedical Research Laboratory, Fort Rucker, AL

The purpose of this investigation was to establish the efficacy of dexedrine for sustaining aviator performance despite 64 hours of extended wakefulness. Although earlier flight studies yielded favorable results with no significant side effects, they were restricted to sleep deprivation periods of only 40 hours. Due to requirements for longer periods of sustained wakefulness, it was necessary to study the efficacy of dexedrine in maintaining aviator performance during 3 days and 2 nights without sleep. To accomplish this, computerized evaluations of aviator flight skills were conducted at regular intervals as subjects completed standardized flights in a UH-60 helicopter simulator, under both dexedrine and placebo. Laboratory-based assessments of cognitive, psychological, and central nervous system status were completed as well. Dexedrine (10 mg) was given prophylactically (prior to signs of fatigue) at midnight, 0400, and 0800 on both deprivation days in one cycle, and placebo was given on both days in the other.

Results indicated that simulator flight performance was maintained by dexedrine for up to 58 hours, while performance under placebo deteriorated significantly. The drug was most beneficial at 0500 and 0900 on the first deprivation day, but it continued to attenuate impairments throughout 1700 on the second deprivation day (after 58 hours awake). Dexedrine likewise lessened the slowing of response times, the impairments in problem identification, and the reductions in performance capabilities that were evident in the cognitive data under placebo. The positive effects of dexedrine were noticeable after only 22 hours of sustained wakefulness but were most evident between 0500 and 1200 on both deprivation days (the times at which performance under placebo suffered the most). These were the same times at which the differences between dexedrine and placebo were most apparent in the flight data. Dexedrine suppressed the increases in slow-wave electroencephalogram (EEG) activity (associated with impaired alertness), which began to occur under the placebo condition after 23 hours of continuous wakefulness. The medication then attenuated a further increase in slow EEG activity that was present throughout 55 hours (and sometimes 59 hours) of deprivation. At the same time, dexedrine (compared to placebo) clearly sustained self-perceptions of vigor, alertness, energy, and talkativeness, while reducing problems with fatigue, confusion, and sleepiness. Mood declines were observed after 20 hours without sleep under the placebo condition, and these were followed by further decrements that were most noticeable after 48 hours of continuous wakefulness. Ratings actually improved under dexedrine at several times. Recovery sleep was slightly less restful under dexedrine even though the last dose was 15 hours before bedtime (dexedrine has an average half-life of 10.25 hours). Thus, at least two nights of recovery sleep should be required after dexedrine is used to delay sleep for 64 hours.

There were no clinically significant side effects that led to the discontinuation of any participant; however, one subject experienced an increase in diastolic blood pressure that would have been cause for concern had it not decreased when the subject was retested in a prone position. Some aviators complained of palpitations and "jitteriness" under dexedrine, but this did not detract from their performance. One of the subjects became very excitable and talkative under the influence of dexedrine, but he did not become reckless or dangerous.

In summary, prophylactic dexedrine administration substantially reduced the impact of sleep loss in the early morning hours and, for the most part, preserved performance for the remainder of the day in a 64-hour bout of continuous wakefulness. The beneficial effects of dexedrine are most apparent during the circadian trough where performance and alertness under placebo are the worst. Thus, when proper restorative sleep is not available due to operational constraints, dexedrine should be considered an effective countermeasure; however, it should not be used as a substitute for sleep. Proper crew rest management must remain a top priority to preserve our tactical advantage on the battlefield.

EFFECT OF NAPS AND CAFFEINE ON ALERTNESS DURING SLEEP LOSS AND NOCTURNAL WORK PERIODS

M.H. Bonnet, Ph.D. and D.L. Arand, Ph.D.
Dayton Department of Veterans Affairs Medical Center, Wright State University, and Kettering Medical Center, Dayton, OH

This work was performed at the Long Beach Veterans Administration Medical Center and the San Diego Naval Health Research Center and supported by a Merit Review Grant from the Department of Veterans Affairs, the Sleep–Wake Disorders Research Institute, and the Naval Medical Research and Development Command, Department of the Navy, Bethesda, Maryland, under Research Work Unit 61153N MR. 04101-03-6003. The views presented in this paper are those of the authors. No endorsement by the Department of the Navy has been given or should be inferred.

Methods

Three studies involving 176 male college students or naval recruits have examined alertness and performance over extended periods of sleep loss. Subjects were chosen to be in good health, to have normal sleep habits, and to be moderate daily caffeine users (250 mg or less). In the first study, groups either (1) went for 64 hours with no sleep or caffeine, (2) had prophylactic naps of 2, 4, or 8 hours prior to sleep loss, or (3) received caffeine at 150, 300, or 400 mg during sleep loss. In the second study, subjects had a 4-hour prophylactic nap prior to sleep loss and then additionally received caffeine at 200 mg (eleveine) during the night. In the third study, subjects either had a 4-hour prophylactic nap prior to sleep loss and received 200 mg of caffeine (eleveine) during the night or had four 1-hour naps during the night.

Results

The results of the first study showed a dose–response effect for length of prophylactic nap and caffeine. Alertness and performance during sleep loss were significantly improved compared to the placebo no-nap group. Alertness was increased most by 8 hours of sleep. The improvement after caffeine use was more similar to that seen after 2–4 hours of additional sleep, except that the effects of caffeine were limited by its metabolic half-life. None of the interventions were able to overcome the profound loss of alertness on the second night of sleep deprivation. The results of the second study indicated that the beneficial effects of caffeine and prophylactic naps were additive (i.e., a prophylactic nap followed by nocturnal use of caffeine left nocturnal alertness and performance at daytime baseline levels). The third study showed that a prophylactic nap followed by nocturnal use of caffeine was superior in maintaining nocturnal performance compared to a series of nocturnal naps, perhaps because the nocturnal naps resulted in sleep inertia.

B

Previous Recommendations on Caffeine from the Committee on Military Nutrition Research

The following is an excerpt from: Institute of Medicine. 1994. *Food Compontents to Enhance Performance.* Washington, DC: National Academy Press. Pp. 32–34, 56–57.

CAFFEINE

The literature on the effects of caffeine on behavior, performance, and health is extensive and somewhat contradictory (for reviews see, for example, Bergman and Dews, 1987; Graham 1987; Hughes et al., 1988; Jarvis, 1993; Smith et al., 1994a,b). David Penetar and colleagues (chapter 20) present a new study on the effects of caffeine on cognitive performance, mood, and alertness in human subjects who had been sleep-deprived, and summarize current knowledge about the use of such supplements. Caffeine is known to exert its central nervous system-mediated effects by blockade of adenosine receptors. Its stimulant effects when compared with those of other drugs such as amphetamines are weak, but most studies to date suggest that it tends to delay sleep, reduce the deterioration of performance associated with fatigue and boredom, and decrease steadiness of the hands, particularly when performance is already partially degraded by repetitive, nonintellectual tasks.

Less well understood are the effects of caffeine in reversing changes caused by sleep deprivation. To clarify these issues, three doses of caffeine (150, 300, and 600 mg/70 kg of body weight) were assessed among normal healthy males after 2 days of sleep deprivation. Cognitive performance, mood, alertness, vital signs, serum caffeine concentrations, and plasma catecholamine levels were also assessed.

Cognitive performance was measured using a computerized assessment battery. Choice reaction time (for 8 hours) significantly improved after caffeine administration, although tests of code substitution and immediate and delayed recall were unaffected.

Mood was assessed by ratings on a profile of mood states questionnaire. Significant increases in vigor were reported for 2 hours after taking the dose, with decreases in fatigue and confusion. Also, significant improvements in mood for 2 hours postdose were reported on visual analog scales for increased alertness, confidence, energy level, and talkativeness and decreased sleepiness. However, anxiety and jitteryness/nervousness also increased. At 12 hours postadministration, ratings for increased energy levels, decreased sleepiness, and jitteryness/nervousness remained elevated.

Alertness, assessed by the modified multiple sleep latency test, also improved for 4.5 hours after caffeine administration, returning to 50 percent of rested levels when the highest doses were used. Oral body temperature remained elevated for 12 hours and blood pressure (diastolic) for one hour, but neither rate nor systolic blood pressure were elevated.

It was concluded that large doses of caffeine reversed sleep deprivation-induced degradation in cognitive performance, mood, and alertness without serious side effects. These data were consistent with those represented in most other studies reviewed. Therefore, Penetar et al. (Chapter 20) recommended that caffeine be included in rations at 250 mg per tablet and that it be made available to soldiers for maintaining performance during specific military operations. The authors did not study individuals with habitually high levels of caffeine ingestion; it would be useful to determine whether the effects of the doses of 300–600 mg noted in this study were as pronounced in individuals with markedly higher levels of typical intakes.

Sustaining optimal soldier performance is recognized to depend on other measures as well. The first is training, so that tasks can be performed with a minimal level of cognitive effort, cross-training so that individuals can substitute for each other, developing and adhering to appropriate work and rest cycles, exercising wise leadership so that unnecessary demands are not placed on subordinates, and modification of systems to minimize errors. Second is enforcing sleep discipline so that the sleep-deprived individual sleeps as much as he or she can and in as hygienic a manner as possible.

The relationship between caffeine intake and health outcomes, particularly cancer incidence, cardiovascular disease (CVD), and effects on fertility, and pregnancy and child outcome, has been the focus of many studies. While data from individual studies have been contradictory, reviews tend to conclude that there is no significant association or negligible/transient effects relating moderate caffeine consumption and cancer, CVD, fertility, and osteoporosis (see, for example, AMAC, 1984; Cooper et al., 1992; Gordis, 1990; Joesoef et al., 1990; Johansson et al., 1992; Lubin and Ron, 1990; Olsen, 1991; Rosenberg, 1990; Schairer et al., 1986; Wilson et al., 1989). However, reports continue to demonstrate that caffeine intake causes an elevation in blood pressure (Smith et al., 1994a,b). Although the blood pressure elevation produced by caffeine has been interpreted as transient and within the range produced by typical activities

(HHS, 1988; Myers, 1988), blood pressure bears monitoring in any future studies of performance enhancement with caffeine supplementation. Recent reports that assess the safety of caffeine consumption during pregnancy have continued to produce conflicting information (Eskenazi, 1993; Infante-Rivard et al., 1993; Mills et al., 1993). These data indicate that high levels of caffeine intake (> 300 mg/d) potentially increase the risk of spontaneous abortion and intrauterine growth retardation during pregnancy (Mills et al;, 1993). The risk to pregnant women of low levels of caffeine intake is uncertain. Further, women often do not realize they are pregnant and/or do not receive prenatal care until after the time period when most spontaneous abortions occur. Should the Army pursue further research in performance enhancement using caffeine products, these health issues must be carefully considered.

In summary, continued research on the mechanisms for the evident effects of caffeine on cognitive performance, mood, and alertness and how these may be enhanced in combination with other dietary measures is warranted. Of particular interest is how to maximize positive effects when performance is already degraded. Individual differences, expectancy, and placebo effects need further elucidation. In the meantime, practical applications of demonstrated effects in ration planning may be in order.

COMMITTEE RECOMMENDATIONS REGARDING FOOD COMPONENTS PROPOSED BY THE ARMY

1. The following components have clearly demonstrated their ability to enhance performance under appropriate simulated conditions and should be evaluated in appropriate delivery systems.

Caffeine. Caffeine functions as a weak stimulant that, in low doses, tends to delay sleep and reduce the deterioration of performance associated with fatigue and boredom. At higher doses caffeine reverses the sleep deprivation-induced degradation in cognitive performance, mood, and alertness. The long experience with the use of coffee suggests that caffeine is safe at levels required to achieve the desired effects, and its effects are reversible over time. **The primary issues that need to be answered in providing caffeine are the appropriate carrier that should be used to provide the supplement and the amount required to achieve the desired benefit in those both habituated and nonhabituated to it.** Since it would not be desirable to inhibit sleep when operations permit, the timing of ingestion and availability of the caffeine-containing food component should be evaluated.

C

Biographical Sketches

COMMITTEE

JOHN E. VANDERVEEN (*Chair*) is the former director of the Food and Drug Administration's (FDA) Office of Plant and Dairy Foods and Beverages in Washington, D.C. His previous position at the FDA was director of the Division of Nutrition at the Center for Food Safety and Applied Nutrition. He also served in various capacities at the U.S. Air Force School of Aerospace Medicine at Brooks Air Force Base, Texas. He has received accolades for service from the FDA and the Air Force. Dr. Vanderveen is a member of the American Society for Clinical Nutrition, American Institute of Nutrition, Aerospace Medical Association, American Dairy Science Association, and the American Chemical Society; a fellow of the Institute of Food Technologists; and an honorary member of the American Dietetic Association. He has served as the treasurer of the American Society of Clinical Nutrition and as a member of the Institute of Food Technology's National Academy of Sciences Advisory Committee. Dr. Vanderveen holds a B.S. in agriculture from Rutgers University in New Jersey and a Ph.D. in chemistry from the University of New Hampshire.

LAWRENCE E. ARMSTRONG is an associate professor of exercise science at the University of Connecticut. He has joint appointments in the Department of Physiology and Neurobiology and the Department of Nutritional Sciences. Dr. Armstrong received his Ph.D. in human bioenergetics–exercise physiology from Ball State University. His research interests include thermoregulation, fluid-electrolyte balance, energy metabolism, exercise physiology, and the human heat illnesses. He previously served as a research physiologist at the U.S. Army Research Institute of Environmental Medicine. He is a fellow of the American search Institute of Environmental Medicine. He is a fellow of the American College of Sports Medicine and a member of the Federation of American Societies for Experimental Biology and the Aerospace Medical Association.

GAIL E. BUTTERFIELD was director of nutrition research for Palo Alto Veterans Affairs Health Care System in California; a lecturer in the Department of Medicine, Stanford University Medical School; visiting assistant professor in the Program of Human Biology, Stanford University; and director of nutrition in the Program in Sports Medicine, Stanford University Medical School. Her previous academic appointments were at the University of California, Berkeley. Dr. Butterfield belonged to the American Institute of Nutrition, American Society for Clinical Nutrition, American Dietetic Association, and American Physiological Society. She was a fellow of the American College of Sports Medicine (ACSM), served as chair of the Pronouncements Committee, and was on the ACSM Board of Trustees; she also was president and executive director of the southwest chapter of that organization. She was a member of the Respiratory and Applied Physiology Study Section of the National Institutes of Health and had served on the editorial boards of the following journals: *Medicine and Science in Sports and Exercise, American Journal of Clinical Nutrition, Health and Fitness Journal of ACSM, Canadian Journal of Clinical Sports Medicine,* and *International Journal of Sports Nutrition.* Dr. Butterfield received her A.B. in biological sciences, M.A. in anatomy, and M.S. and Ph.D. in nutrition from the University of California, Berkeley. Her research interests included nutrition in exercise, effect of growth factors on protein metabolism in the elderly, and metabolic fuel use in women exposed to high altitude. She died suddenly on December 27, 1999.

WANDA L. CHENOWETH is a professor in the Department of Food Science and Human Nutrition at Michigan State University. Previously, she held positions as teaching associate at the University of Iowa and University of California, Berkeley. Other work experience includes positions as research dietitian and head clinical dietitian at University of Iowa Hospitals and as research dietitian at the Mayo Clinic. She is a member of the American Society for Nutritional Sciences, American Dietetic Association, and Institute of Food Technology. She serves as a reviewer for several journals, including the *Journal of the American Dietetic Association, American Journal of Clinical Nutrition,* and *Journal of Nutrition,* and is a member of the Associate Editorial Board of *Plant Foods for Human Nutrition.* She has served on a technical review committee for the Diet, Nutrition, and Cancer Program of the National Cancer Institute and as a site evaluator for the Commission on Evaluation of Dietetic Education of the American Dietetic Association. Her research interests are in the areas of mineral bioavailability and clinical nutrition. Dr. Chenoweth completed a B.S. in dietetics from the University of Iowa, dietetic internship and M.S. in nutrition at the University of Iowa, and a Ph.D. in nutrition at the University of California, Berkeley.

JOHANNA T. DWYER is the director of the Frances Stern Nutrition Center at New England Medical Center, professor of medicine and community health at the Tufts University School of Medicine, and professor of nutrition at Tufts University School of Nutrition in Boston. She is also senior scientist at the Jean Mayer U.S. Department of Agriculture (USDA) Human Nutrition Research Center on Aging at Tufts. Dr. Dwyer is the author or coauthor of more than 100 research articles and 185 review articles published in scientific journals. Her work centers on life-cycle-related concerns such as the prevention of diet-related disease in children and adolescents and maximization of quality of life and health in the elderly. She also has a long-standing interest in vegetarian and other alternative life-styles. Dr. Dwyer is a past president of the American Institute of Nutrition, past secretary of the American Society for Clinical Nutrition, and past president and current fellow of the Society for Nutrition Education. She served on the Program Development Board of the American Public Health Association from 1989 to 1992 and is a former member of the Food and Nutrition Board of the Institute of Medicine, and a member of the Technical Advisory Committee of the Nutrition Screening Initiative, and the Board of Directors of the American Institute of Wine and Food. As a Robert Wood Johnson Health Policy Fellow (1980–1981), she served on the personal staffs of Senator Richard Lugar (R-Indiana) and Senator Barbara Mikulski (D-Maryland). Dr. Dwyer has received numerous honors and awards for her work in the field of nutrition, including the 1996 W.O. Atwater Award of the USDA and the J. Harvey Wiley Award from the Society for Nutrition Education. She gave the Lenna Frances Cooper Lecture at the annual meeting of the American Dietetic Association in 1990. Dr. Dwyer is currently on the editorial boards of *Family Economics* and *Nutrition Review* and the advisory board of *Clinics in Applied Nutrition*; she is a contributing editor to *Nutrition Reviews*, as well as a reviewer for the *Journal of the American Dietetic Association*, *American Journal of Clinical Nutrition*, and *American Journal of Public Health*. She received her D.Sc. and M.Sc. from the Harvard School of Public Health, an M.S. from the University of Wisconsin, and her undergraduate degree with distinction from Cornell University.

JOHN D. FERNSTROM is professor of psychiatry, pharmacology, and behavioral neuroscience at the University of Pittsburgh School of Medicine, and director of the Basic Neuroendocrinology Program at the Western Psychiatric Institute and Clinic. He received his B.S. in biology and his Ph.D. in nutritional biochemistry from the Massachusetts Institute of Technology (MIT). He was a postdoctoral fellow in neuroendocrinology at the Roche Institute for Molecular Biology in Nutley, New Jersey. Before coming to the University of Pittsburgh,

Dr. Fernstrom was an assistant and then associate professor in the Department of Nutrition and Food Science at MIT. He has served on numerous governmental advisory committees. He presently is a member of the National Advisory Council of the Monell Chemical Senses Center, chairman of the Neurosciences Section of the American Society for Nutritional Sciences (ASNS), and a member of the ASNS Council. He is a member of numerous professional societies, including the American Institute of Nutrition, the American Society for Clinical Nutrition, the American Physiological Society, the American Society for Pharmacology and Experimental Therapeutics, the American Society for Neurochemistry, the Society for Neuroscience, and the Endocrine Society. Among other awards, Dr. Fernstrom received the Mead-Johnson Award of the American Institute of Nutrition, a Research Scientist Award from the National Institute of Mental Health, a Wellcome Visiting Professorship in the Basic Medical Sciences, and an Alfred P. Sloan Fellowship in Neurochemistry. His current major research interest concerns the influence of the diet and drugs on the synthesis of neurotransmitters in the central and peripheral nervous systems.

ROBIN B. KANAREK is professor of psychology and professor of nutrition at Tufts University in Medford, Massachusetts, where she also is the chair of the Department of Psychology. Her prior experience includes research fellow, Division of Endocrinology, University of California, Los Angeles School of Medicine, and research fellow in nutrition at Harvard University. In addition to reviewing for several journals, including *Science*, *Brain Research Bulletin*, *Journal of Nutrition*, *American Journal of Clinical Nutrition*, and *Annals of Internal Medicine*, she is a member of the editorial boards of *Physiology and Behavior* and the *Tufts Diet and Nutrition Newsletter* and past editor-in-chief of *Nutrition and Behavior*. Dr. Kanarek has served on ad hoc review committees for the National Science Foundation, National Institutes of Health, and U.S. Department of Agriculture nutrition research, as well as the Member Program Committee of the Eastern Psychological Association. She is a fellow of the American College of Nutrition, and her other professional memberships include the American Institute of Nutrition, New York Academy of Sciences, Society for the Study of Ingestive Behavior, and Society for Neurosciences. Dr. Kanarek received a B.A. in biology from Antioch College in Yellow Springs, Ohio, and an M.S. and Ph.D. in psychology from Rutgers University in New Brunswick, New Jersey.

ORVILLE A. LEVANDER is a research chemist for the U.S. Department of Agriculture (USDA) Nutrient Requirements and Functions Laboratory in the Human Nutrition Research Center in Beltsville, Maryland. He was resident fellow in biochemistry at Colombia University's College of Physicians and Surgeons, and research associate at Harvard University's School of Public Health. Dr. Levander served on the Food and Nutrition Board's Committee on

Dietary Allowances. He also served on panels of the National Research Council's Committees on Animal Nutrition and on the Biological Effects of Environmental Pollutants. He was a member of the U.S. National Committee for the International Union of Nutrition Scientists and temporary adviser to the World Health Organization's Environmental Health Criteria Document on Selenium. Dr. Levander was awarded the Osborne and Mendel Award from the American Institute of Nutrition. His society memberships include the American Institute of Nutrition, American Chemical Society, and American Society for Clinical Nutrition. Dr. Levander received his B.A. from Cornell University and his M.S. and Ph.D. in biochemistry from the University of Wisconsin, Madison.

ESTHER M. STERNBERG is chief of the Section on Neuroendocrine Immunology and Behavior and director of the Integrated Neural Immune Program of the National Institute of Mental Health Intramural Research Program at the National Institutes of Health (NIH). Dr. Sternberg received her M.D. degree and trained in rheumatology at McGill University, Montreal, Canada. She did postdoctoral training at Washington University, Barnes Hospital, St. Louis, Missouri, in the Division of Allergy and Immunology. She was subsequently a Howard Hughes Associate and instructor in the Department of Medicine at Washington University and Barnes Hospital before joining NIH. Dr. Sternberg is internationally recognized for her ground-breaking discoveries in the area of central nervous system–immune system interactions. She has received the Arthritis Foundation William R. Felts Award for Excellence in Rheumatology Research Publications, has been awarded the Public Health Service Superior Service Award, and has been elected to the American Society for Clinical Investigation in recognition of this work. Dr. Sternberg is also internationally recognized as a foremost authority on the L-tryptophan eosinophilia–myalgia syndrome (L-TRP-EMS). She was the first to describe this syndrome in relation to a similar drug L-5-hydroxytryptophan and published this landmark article in the *New England Journal of Medicine* in 1980. She received the Food and Drug Commissioner's citation for her work elucidating the pathogenesis of this syndrome.

MARY I. POOS (*Food and Nutrition Board [FNB] Staff, Study Director*) is project director for the Committee on Military Nutrition Research. She joined the FNB of the Institute of Medicine (IOM) in November 1997. She has been a project director for the National Academy of Sciences since 1990. Prior to officially joining the FNB staff, she served as a project director for the National Research Council's Board on Agriculture for more than seven years, two of which were spent on loan to the FNB. Her work with the FNB includes senior staff officer for the IOM report, *The Program of Research for Military Nursing* and study director for the reports, *A Review of the Department of Defense's Program for Breast Cancer Research* and *Vitamin C Fortification of Food Aid Commodities*. Currently, she also serves as study director to the Subcommittee on Interpretation and Uses of Dietary Reference Intakes. While working with the Board on Agriculture, Dr. Poos was responsible for the Committee on Animal Nutrition and directed the production of seven reports in the *Nutrient Requirements of Domestic Animals* series, including a letter report to the commissioner of the Food and Drug Administration concerning the importance of selenium in animal nutrition. Prior to joining the National Academies she was consultant-owner of Nutrition Consulting Services of Greenfield, Massachusetts; assistant professor in the Department of Veterinary and Animal Sciences at the University of Massachusetts, Amherst; and adjunct assistant professor in the Department of Animal Sciences, University of Vermont. She received her B.S. in biology from Virginia Polytechnic Institute and State University and a Ph.D. in animal sciences (nutrition–biochemistry) from the University of Kentucky; she completed a postdoctoral fellowship in the Department of Animal Sciences Area of Excellence Program at the University of Nebraska. Dr. Poos's areas of research interest include protein and nitrogen metabolism and nutrition–reproduction interactions.

SPEAKERS

MICHAEL H. BONNET is professor of neurology at Wright State University of Medicine in Dayton, Ohio. At the Sleep Laboratory in the Department of Neurology at the Department of Veterans' Affairs Hospital in Dayton, Dr. Bonnet conducts research in the areas of sleep deprivation, sleep fragmentation, and insomnia.

JACK L. BRIGGS is the senior food technologist for the Department of Defense Combat Feeding Program, U.S. Army Soldier and Biological Chemical Command, at the Natick Soldier Center. Previously he held positions as a food scientist for Carnation Co., senior scientist at Lipton, and director of research and development at Brilliant Seafood. He received his master's degree in biochemistry from Colorado State University. In his present position as senior food technologist, he is responsible for planning and conducting applications engineering and development activities for ration components. In addition, he coordinates and advises on special technical problems related to the Department of Defense procurement of operational ration components. Currently, Mr. Briggs is working on the formulation and fabrication of novel foods with performance enhancement potential.

JOHN A. CALDWELL is an experimental psychologist and the director of sustained operations research at the U.S. Army Aeromedical Research Laboratory, where he conducts a variety of research on the performance of helicopter pilots. His studies are aimed at fully understanding the effects of sleep deprivation and aviator fatigue and developing countermeasures for use in the operational aviator environment. He conducts both simulator and in-flight pilot performance studies to enhance the efficiency, safety, and well-being of aviators in sustained operations. His efforts have been published in more than 80 separate articles in peer-reviewed scientific journals and laboratory technical reports. Dr. Caldwell is an adjunct faculty member at the School of Aerospace Medicine and the Aviation Pre Command Course at Fort Rucker, and he frequently lectures at safety briefings and scientific symposia. He is a member of the National Sleep Foundation's Speakers Bureau on operator fatigue and frequently consults with various organizations on the effects of fatigue on pilots and methods for overcoming the adverse impact of fatigue in the aviation environment.

ROLAND R. GRIFFITHS is a professor of behavioral biology and professor of neuroscience at the Johns Hopkins University School of Medicine in Baltimore, Maryland. He received his Ph.D. in psychopharmacology from the University of Minnesota in 1972. Excluding abstracts and short reports, the total number of Dr. Griffiths' publications exceeds 200, and he has published more than 25 articles directly related to caffeine use in humans and caffeine dependence.

STEPHEN G. HOLTZMAN is a professor of pharmacology at Emory University School of Medicine in Atlanta, Georgia. In addition, he holds an appointment as a collaborative scientist in the Division of Neuroscience, Yerkes Regional Primate Research Center at Emory. He received his Ph.D. in pharmacology at the University of Michigan in 1969. Dr. Holtzman has won numerous honors and served on various committees related to drug abuse and dependence.

JOHN L. IVY is professor and coordinator of the Exercise Science Program in the College of Education, Department of Kinesiology and Health, and the College of Pharmacy, Division of Pharmacology, at the University of Texas in Austin. In 1998 he was awarded the Margie Gurley Seay Centennial Professorship. Other honors include a fellowship in the American Academy of Kinesiology and Physical Education, Dean's Fellowship for Excellence in Research, the Judy Spence Frank Endowed Fellowship for Excellence, and membership in Sigma Xi, the Scientific Research Society. Dr. Ivy was associate editor of *Research Quarterly for Exercise and Sports,* and currently serves on the editorial boards of *Medicine and Science in Sports and Exercise, American Journal of Physiology, Endocrinology and Metabolism, Journal of Optimal Nutrition, International Journal of Sports Nutrition,* and *Diabetes Forecast.*

RICHARD F. JOHNSON is a research psychologist in the Military Performance Division at the U.S. Army Research Institute of Environmental Medicine (USARIEM), Natick, Massachusetts. He received his Ph.D. in psychology (1970) from Brandeis University, where he was both a National Aeronautics and Space Administration trainee and a Woodrow Wilson dissertation fellow. Prior to joining USARIEM in 1984, he served as a captain in the U.S. Army Medical

Service Corps (1970–1972), was a National Institute of Mental Health grantee (1972–1976), and was a research psychologist with the U.S. Army Natick Research and Development Laboratories (1976–1983). He is a senior lecturer in psychology at Northeastern University and has published in the areas of psychophysiology, experimental research methodology, and stress. He is a fellow of both the American Psychological Association and the American Psychological Society, and is a past president of the Natick Chapter of Sigma Xi, the Scientific Research Society. His current research interests include the effects of environmental extremes and military operational demands on vigilance, psychomotor behavior, and subjective response.

GARY H. KAMIMORI is a research physiologist in the Department of Neurobiology and Behavior, Division of Neuropsychiatry, at Walter Reed Army Institute of Research.

MARY A. KAUTZ has been a research psychologist in the Department of Neurobiology and Behavior, Division of Neuropsychiatry, at the Walter Reed Army Institute of Research (WRAIR) since January 1998. She came on active duty as a direct commissioned officer in October 1997. She holds a Ph.D. in experimental psychology from the American University in Washington, D.C., and has completed two postdoctoral fellowships—one at Johns Hopkins University School of Medicine and a second at Bowman Gray School of Medicine of Wake Forest University. Her interests prior to coming on active duty included behavioral psychopharmacology research with benzodiazapines and alcohol in nonhuman primates. While at WRAIR, her research focus has been on determining militarily relevant relationships between variables, including physiological measures of brain activity, sleep, arousal, cognitive performance, and drugs (particularly stimulants as they are used to enhance cognitive performance following extended periods of sleep deprivation).

HARRIS R. LIEBERMAN is deputy chief of the Military Nutrition and Biochemistry Division of the U.S. Army Research Institute of Environmental Medicine (USARIEM) in Natick, Massachusetts. Dr. Lieberman is an internationally recognized expert in the area of nutrition and behavior and has published more than 90 original, full-length papers in scientific journals and edited books. He has been an invited lecturer at numerous national and international conferences, government research laboratories, and universities. Dr. Lieberman received his Ph.D. in physiological psychology in 1977 from the University of Florida. Upon completing his graduate training he was awarded a National Institutes of Health fellowship to conduct postdoctoral research at the Department of Psychology and Brain Science at the Massachusetts Institute of Technology (MIT). In 1980 he was appointed to the research staff at MIT and established an interdisciplinary research program in the Department of Brain and Cognitive Sciences to examine the effects of various food constituents and drugs on human behavior and brain function. Key accomplishments of the laboratory included the development of appropriate methods for assessing the effects of food constituents and other subtle environmental factors on human brain function and the determination that specific foods and hormones reliably alter human performance. In 1990 Dr. Lieberman joined the civilian research staff of USARIEM where he has continued his work in nutrition and behavior. He has addressed the effects of various nutritional factors, diets, and environmental stress on animal and human performance, brain function, and behavior. His research program has focused on developing and applying a variety of emerging technologies to sustaining and enhancing human performance.

DAVID M. PENETAR currently is the commander of the U.S. Army Research Institute of Environmental Medicine, Natick, Massachusetts. He earned his Ph.D. in psychopharmacology from the University of Minnesota in 1977. His research experience includes the assessment of sleep deprivation and caffeine effects on cognitive performance conducted while assigned to the Walter Reed Army Institute of Research.

W.K. PRUSACZYK received his B.A. and M.S. degrees in psychology and his Ph.D. in exercise physiology from the University of Georgia. He then went on active duty in the U.S. Army and was stationed at the U.S. Army Research Institute of Environmental Medicine in Natick, Massachusetts. After serving three years in the Military Ergonomics Division, Dr. Prusaczyk left active duty and began work at the Naval Health Research Center (NHRC), San Diego, California. While at NHRC his early work focused on thermoregulation and thermal protection systems for Naval Sea–Air–Land (SEAL) personnel. After five years of work in the field with SEALs, Dr. Prusaczyk assumed the position of head, Applied Physiology Division, in the Human Performance Department at NHRC, managing broad research projects in thermal physiology, occupational physiology, and body composition. In 1997 Dr. Prusaczyk was promoted to head, Human Performance Department. His current research interests are in thermal physiology and protective systems, occupational physiology, and performance enhancement methodologies.

CHRISTINE SCHLICTING is from the Naval Submarine Medical Research Laboratory at the Naval Submarine Base, New London, Connecticut.

ANDREW SMITH is professor of experimental psychology and director of the Health Psychology Research Unit, University of Bristol. He did his undergraduate and Ph.D. work at University College in London. He conducted postdoctoral research at Oxford University from 1976 to 1982. He then worked for the Medical Research Council at Sussex University from 1982 to 1988 and was a reader at University of Wales College of Cardiff from 1990 to 1993 before taking up his current post at Bristol. He has published widely in the areas of nutrition and behavior, with one of his main interests being the effects of caffeine on performance in low-alertness situations. His research is supported by research councils, government agencies, and industry.

STEVEN R. SMITH graduated from the University of Texas at Arlington in 1984 and the University of Texas Medical School in San Antonio in 1988. He went on to take a residency at Baylor University Medical Center in Dallas and a fellowship in endocrinology at the Ochsner Clinic in New Orleans. He moved to the Pennington Biomedical Research Center in 1994 as an instructor to work on projects sponsored by the National Aeronautics and Space Administration and the Department of Defense. He joined the faculty in 1995 and currently acts as director of the Inpatient Metabolic Unit at the Pennington Center at the level of assistant professor. Dr. Smith's research program includes basic research into the molecular mechanisms of insulin resistance and insulin signaling, clinical studies of energy balance and macronutrient oxidation, and impact of body fat and body fat distribution on the complications of obesity.

LAWRENCE L. SPRIET is a professor in the Department of Human Biology and Nutritional Sciences at the University of Guelph in Guelph, Ontario, Canada. He teaches undergraduate and graduate courses in skeletal muscle metabolism, as well as graduate courses in human muscle metabolism, nutrition, and exercise. Dr. Spriet's research employs both animal and human models to examine the biochemical regulation of the interaction between fat and carbohydrate metabolism in skeletal muscle following dietary interventions and during exercise. Much of this work examines key regulatory enzymes that control the flux through the pathways that produce energy during exercise. His work is supported by funding from the Natural Sciences and Engineering Research Council of Canada. Dr. Spriet is a member of the American and Canadian Physiological Society, American College of Sports Medicine, and Canadian Society for Exercise Physiology.

ROBERT STICKGOLD received his doctoral training in biochemistry at the University of Wisconsin, Madison, and postdoctoral training at Stanford and Harvard Medical Schools. His research has ranged from the enzymology of bacterial cell wall synthesis to analysis of the formal properties of rapid eye movement sleep dreams. For the last 10 years, Dr. Stickgold has focused on the state-dependent aspects of cognition, studying how cognitive functions are altered during sleep, as a consequence of sleep, and in the absence of sleep. His recent work has focused on the critical role of sleep in memory consolidation and integration, as well as on physiological measurements of vigilance.

HANS VAN DONGEN earned his Ph.D. in physiology in 1998 at Leiden University in the Netherlands and is currently a research assistant professor in the Division of Sleep and Chronobiology at the University of Pennsylvania School of Medicine in Philadelphia. He has published widely on the subject of biological rhythms and sleep patterns. He is a member of several professional societies concerned with sleep research and chronobiology, and has served as a reviewer for the journal *Sleep*.

JAMES K. WYATT is an instructor of medicine at Harvard Medical School and associate psychologist at Brigham and Women's Hospital in Boston. He received his Ph.D. in clinical psychology at the University of Arizona in Tucson in 1995. He is a member of the American Psychology Association, American Sleep Disorders Association, Sleep Research Society, and American Association for the Advancement of Science. In addition, Dr. Wyatt is a reviewer for *Sleep*.